The
Glycemic
LOAD
Diet

The Glycemic LOAD Diet

Lose Weight and Balance Blood Sugar with This Powerful New Program

Rob Thompson, MD, with Dana Carpender

RODALE.

Portions of this book were previously published by McGraw Hill as
The Glycemic Load Diet © 2006 by Robert Thompson and *The Glycemic Load Diet
Cookbook* © 2009 by Dana Carpender and Robert Thompson. Exclusive direct mail
edition published by Rodale Inc. in August 2011 under license from McGraw Hill.
© 2006, 2009, 2011 by Robert Thompson.

Printed in the United States of America
Rodale Inc. makes every effort to use acid-free ♾, recycled paper ♻.

Library of Congress Cataloging-in-Publication Data is on file with the publisher.

ISBN 13: 978–1–60961–053–1
4 6 8 10 9 7 5   hardcover

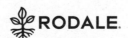

We inspire and enable people to improve their lives and the world around them.
For more of our products visit **rodalestore.com** or call 800-848-4735

To Kathy, Maggie, John, and "Nan"

Contents

Part 2

THE GLYCEMIC LOAD DIET
AND SLOW-TWITCH MUSCLE ACTIVATION PLAN

Acknowledgments

I am indebted to my now-retired agent, Elizabeth Frost-Knappman, for her interest, her encouragement, and her assistance in shepherding this book through its early stages. I would like to thank my editors, Andrea Au Levitt and Bridget Doherty, and their colleagues at Rodale for coming up with the idea of combining *The Glycemic Load* and *The Glycemic Load Cookbook* into a single volume. I also owe thanks to my agent, Roger Williams, for doing an excellent job with the business end.

I owe much to my outstanding office staff, Shannon Pagan and Nadine Warner, for making my life manageable. Most of all, I would like to thank my wife, Kathy, for her unwavering patience, encouragement, and support.

Introduction

When I started practicing medicine 30 years ago, I followed the party line. I recommended calorie counting and low-fat diets for weight loss and was usually disappointed by the results. People just kept gaining weight. Then, in the 1990s, some of my patients started ignoring warnings about fat and cholesterol and going on low-carb diets. The results were astonishing. Folks who had been unsuccessful at losing weight for years started shedding pounds more easily than they thought possible even as they ate generous amounts of rich food. Remarkably, their blood cholesterol and sugar levels looked better than ever. It was as if they had stopped ingesting a toxin that had been poisoning them for years. I became convinced that the low-carbohydrate approach had tremendous potential for helping people lose weight and regain their health. Indeed, as additional research has come out, the medical establishment, mired in low-fat orthodoxy for decades, has come around to thinking the same way.

But just when medical science is focusing more attention on carbohydrates, the public's interest in low-carb diets is waning. People rushed to try the Atkins Diet—a radical low-carb regimen popularized in the 1970s—and the South Beach Diet, a sort of second-generation Atkins Diet, but the programs didn't work the way they hoped. People lost weight but usually gained it back. Although these diets allowed plenty of rich food, they created irresistible food cravings. People just couldn't continue them for long. Disillusionment set in, and the low-carb craze began to die down.

In recent years, billions of dollars have been spent researching human body chemistry. Medical science knows much more about carbohydrate metabolism now than it did when the low-carb movement began such as:

- Food scientists have developed a way of measuring the metabolic effects of different carbohydrates, called the *glycemic index*. This concept, only in its infancy when the low-carb movement began, has evolved into a powerful model, the glycemic load. This new way of looking at carbohydrates radically changes the low-carb approach to losing weight. It is the key to a natural weight-loss-promoting eating style that is satisfying and easy enough to follow for life.
- Scientists now know that most overweight people have a genetically influenced metabolic disorder called *insulin resistance* that makes them susceptible to weight gain from eating carbohydrates with high glycemic loads. Researchers have pinpointed the foods and behavior patterns that exacerbate this condition and can now target treatment toward relieving it.
- Recently, physiologists have discovered the metabolic quirk that causes insulin resistance. It's a disorder of the body's slow-twitch muscle fibers. What's exciting is that exercising these muscle fibers creates much less fatigue than exercising others.

These and other new concepts can help you harness the weight-loss power of carbohydrate modification and slow-twitch muscle activation with a lifestyle that's much easier to follow than previous weight-loss regimens. It really is possible to lose weight without "dieting," in the usual sense of the word, or engaging in strenuous exercise.

Over the years that I've worked with people trying to lose weight, I have developed a sense of what people are capable of. I am convinced that willpower is not a prerequisite for success and, in fact, can be a liability. When it comes to losing weight, we all have limited supplies of energy and discipline. What's critical is finding the right strategy, and the key is knowledge. If you come to understand the physiological disturbances that caused you to gain weight, you will know exactly what you need to do to lose it. Indeed, once you see the light, I think you'll find that shedding pounds and keeping them off for good are much easier than you thought.

Part 1

Insulin Resistance:
A Hormonal
Imbalance, Not a
Character Defect

1

Understanding Why You Gained Weight

I t's enough to drive you crazy. You're constantly battling your weight while others you know seem to stay thin effortlessly. They don't exercise, they eat anything they want, but they don't get fat. The perplexing thing about the obesity epidemic—and this has been true of other scourges throughout history—is that some people are more vulnerable than others. They suffer from the harmful effects of our modern lifestyle, while others seem to be immune. Overeating and lack of exercise are not the whole story.

But for years, people thought that being overweight was a matter of choice. Just as some folks played golf or did crossword puzzles for enjoyment, others got their kicks from eating. Doctors knew of certain hormonal disturbances that could make people gain weight, but they thought these were unusual. They figured that most overweight people just chose to be the way they were.

Of course, who in their right mind would choose to be fat? If it came to a decision between being overweight or getting hit by a truck, some people would probably opt for the truck. Almost everyone would agree: Obesity is unattractive, cumbersome, and unhealthy.

3

Being overweight, then, suggested either you were weak willed or you had some kind of psychological problem. However, when psychologists got around to studying overweight people systematically, they came up empty-handed. It turns out that overweight people are psychologically no different from thin folks. They have some bad habits, but no more than anybody else. One thing is certain: They aren't weak willed. Obese people often show remarkable self-discipline in other aspects of their lives. After all, 65 percent of Americans are overweight. Do all of these people have some kind of character defect? Of course not.

It's Not a Matter of Willpower

Do you remember when you were a kid and you tried to see how long you could hold your breath? It was easy at first, but after a minute or so, you developed a different mind-set. Lack of oxygen triggered chemical reflexes that told you in no uncertain terms you needed to breathe. Certainly, the need for oxygen is more urgent than the need for food, but the principle is the same. If you reduce your caloric intake, changes in your body chemistry stimulate powerful hunger-driving reflexes that overrule lesser concerns—like how good you look. When those instincts say "eat," unless you have unusual willpower, you eat. You can postpone it for a while—and you have some control over the *kinds* of foods you eat—but if you try to defy the urge, you usually come away the loser.

The reason self-deprivation rarely works for losing weight is that it defies deeply rooted survival instincts. Your body has its own systems for regulating your weight, and these mechanisms are largely out of your conscious control. Consider this: Your body burns about 1.2 million calories a year. If your weight depended on your consciously regulating the amount you eat, misjudging by 2 percent (that's about two bites of a potato a day) would add or take off 42 pounds in 10 years. Who can fine-tune their eating that much? Your body can't afford to rely on your whims. It has its own mechanisms for balancing calorie intake with energy output. Just as a lack of willpower didn't make you gain weight, simply willing yourself to eat less is unlikely to result in lasting weight loss. You might think you can dial down your calorie consumption at will, and maybe you can for a while. But let's face it: If you're like most people, those survival instincts will win in the end.

A Matter of Hormones

In recent years, scientists who study body chemistry have discovered several hormones that regulate body weight. Here are a few examples.

- The *beta cells* of your pancreas make *insulin,* a powerful hormone that, among other things, drives calories into your fat stores.
- Your thyroid gland makes a hormone called *thyroxin,* which helps regulate how fast your body burns calories.
- Your stomach secretes *ghrelin* to stimulate your appetite when your stomach is empty.
- Your intestines produce *peptide YY* to curb your appetite when your intestines have enough food to work on.
- Your fat cells secrete *leptin* to reduce your appetite when your fat stores have been replenished.

These are only some of the hormones known to control weight, and scientists are still discovering new ones. The point is this: Powerful chemical reflexes regulate the balance between the calories you take in and the rate at which you burn them. Body weight is not simply a matter of choice.

The hormone systems that regulate body weight evolved over millions of years during times when hunger was a constant threat. Although these mechanisms helped keep fat accumulation in check, their main purpose was to prevent starvation. While our lifestyles have changed a lot since the Stone Age, our body chemistries work the same. When our weight-regulating systems sense we're not getting enough to eat, hunger-stimulating hormones arouse powerful cravings, and energy-regulating hormones reduce the rate at which our bodies burn calories. The desire to eat dominates our thoughts, and our bodies do everything they can to replenish fat.

So the reason you're overweight is not that you lack willpower. It's because something upset the systems that match your caloric intake with your energy expenditure. Certainly, choices were involved. You influenced the *form* those calories took—whether they were carbohydrates, fats, or protein—but your body's weight-regulating mechanisms determined how much food you needed to quell your hunger. You can't ignore those instincts. Mustering up the discipline to starve yourself is not the answer.

But if you have such little control over how much you eat, how can you lose weight? It's actually easier than you think, but you just can't do it by a frontal assault on deeply rooted survival instincts.

There are dozens of ways to lose weight. You can cut fats, cut carbs, count calories, fast, go on an exercise kick, or have your stomach stapled. But if a particular problem—say a hormonal imbalance, a lifestyle quirk, or a certain kind of food—caused you to gain weight, does it make sense to just starve yourself without trying to correct the conditions that caused the problem in the first place? If you don't fix what's wrong, whatever caused you to put on the pounds is bound to come back to haunt you. You need to know *why* you gained weight.

Unlocking the Mystery of Obesity

In recent years, billions of dollars have been spent on researching human metabolism, and indeed, medical science has made major breakthroughs in solving the mystery of obesity. Although these advances have been obscured by the usual academic squabbling, junk science, and advertising hype that surround the issue of weight loss, new scientific discoveries have turned old ways of thinking upside down. Scientists now have a clearer idea of why people's weight-regulating mechanisms fall out of kilter and what can be done to put them back in balance. Here is the picture that is emerging.

If you're like most overweight people, three conditions converged to cause you to gain weight.

1. You have a common genetic quirk that affects a type of muscle fiber in your body called *slow-twitch fibers,* causing

them to fall into a deeper-than-normal dormant state when you don't use them.

2. Lack of regular activation of your slow-twitch fibers causes them to lose sensitivity to insulin, a hormone needed to metabolize the sugar glucose. This condition is called *insulin resistance*. Because of loss of sensitivity to insulin, your body has to produce greater-than-normal amounts of insulin to handle *carbohydrates*—foods your digestive tract breaks down into glucose.

3. The insensitivity of your muscles to insulin makes you vulnerable to the harmful effects of dietary *starch*—the main ingredient of carbohydrate staples such as bread, potatoes, and rice—and sugar. Starch and sugar release more glucose into your bloodstream and do it faster than other kinds of food.

Here's what happens: If your muscles are resistant to insulin and you consume quantities of starch and sugar typical of our modern diet, your beta cells have to make as much as *five or six times* the normal amount of insulin to handle the glucose in your blood. And that's the problem. Insulin is a powerful obesity-promoting hormone.

As it turns out, small amounts of insulin actually suppress appetite and *prevent* overeating. However, excessive amounts drive calories into your fat stores and virtually lock them in so your body can't use them for energy. Scientists call this "internal starvation." It creates the frustrating paradox of obesity: Even though you have plenty of calories stored up as fat, you're hungry all the time. Excessive insulin makes you want to eat more than you need and encourages your body to store calories as fat. Try as you will, you can't keep the pounds off.

There's another problem with starch and sugar: Instead of traversing the full 22 feet of your digestive tract as other foods do, they short-circuit into your bloodstream in the first foot or two. They never reach the last part of your intestine, where certain appetite-suppressing hormones come from—another reason why, even though starch and sugar are chock-full of calories, a few hours after eating them, you're hungry again.

Sleuthing the Hormonal Culprit: Syndrome X

Doctors have known for years that certain diseases can throw people's weight-regulating mechanisms out of kilter. The best known of these conditions is hypothyroidism, an underactive thyroid gland. Many folks wish they had hypothyroidism because it's so easy to correct with pills. However, most people's weight problems are not caused by thyroid trouble.

Although doctors have known for years of conditions that cause unwanted weight gain in the occasional patient, until recently they couldn't pinpoint what caused *most* cases of obesity. Whatever it was, though, it was apparent that it was extremely common and the modern lifestyle aggravated it. Then scientists got a clue from doctors who take care of heart patients.

In the 1980s, some doctors noticed that patients who'd suffered heart attacks had an unusually high incidence of the following physical characteristics and laboratory findings:

- Visceral adiposity, a tendency to accumulate fat in the abdomen
- High blood levels of a type of fat called *triglyceride*
- Low blood levels of HDL, a protective kind of cholesterol particle also called "good cholesterol"
- Mildly elevated blood pressure
- Borderline-high blood glucose levels

When several of those findings occurred in the same individual, it raised the risk of heart attack *even when blood cholesterol levels were normal.* Not knowing what caused this phenomenon, doctors called it "syndrome X" or "the metabolic syndrome."

It didn't take long for scientists to figure out what causes the metabolic syndrome: It's brought on by the combination of insulin resistance and excessive consumption of starch and sugar. This discovery turned the nutrition world upside down and invalidated much of what doctors previously believed about diet, obesity, and heart disease. It also explained why excessive dietary starch and sugar, along with a lack of physical activity, have led to an epidemic of diabetes and obesity.

Insulin Resistance: A Late-Twentieth-Century Scourge

Insulin resistance isn't exactly a disease—it's a common variation in the way people's bodies process carbohydrates, foods your body breaks down into glucose. About 22 percent of the American population can't handle the starch and sugar in their diets without producing excessive insulin, which puts them at risk of obesity and other hallmarks of the metabolic syndrome. Although these individuals usually have a genetic propensity to insulin resistance, having the tendency doesn't necessarily bring on the condition. People who are hereditarily predisposed can go their entire lives without gaining unhealthy amounts of weight or manifesting other signs of the metabolic syndrome. Something else—something in their activity and eating patterns—has to bring it on.

Insulin resistance is not a problem of some internal organ, such as your liver or your kidneys; it's basically a problem with your muscles. They are the main users of glucose, and the target of most of the insulin your body produces. Exercise increases your muscles' responsiveness to insulin, and inactivity decreases their sensitivity. While the lack of physical activity that characterizes the typical modern lifestyle causes some degree of insulin resistance in everybody, it renders the muscles of genetically prone individuals particularly insensitive to insulin.

Although lack of physical activity brings on insulin resistance, this wouldn't be a problem if we ate only meat and raw vegetation, as our prehistoric ancestors did. Your body doesn't need much insulin to handle those foods. Meat contains virtually no glucose, and the glucose in fresh fruit and vegetables trickles into your bloodstream slowly, requiring only small amounts of insulin. The only foods in our diet that call for large amounts of insulin are so-called refined carbohydrates such as flour products, potatoes, rice, and sweets. Insulin resistance becomes a problem only when you consume more starch and sugar than your body can handle.

There's another important factor that brings on insulin resistance: being overweight itself. It's a vicious cycle. Weight gain worsens insulin resistance, and insulin resistance, in turn, promotes more weight gain. Even if you weren't insulin resistant to begin with, if you're overweight, you're more insulin resistant now than you were before. If you continue consuming the same amount of starch and sugar as you did before, you will have to produce more insulin than you did before to handle it, which makes losing weight increasingly difficult.

The Thrifty-Gene Hypothesis

Why are so many of us genetically prone to such a troublesome condition as obesity? One benefit of being overweight is that you can withstand starvation better than thinner folks can. In ancient times, when humans regularly went long periods without food, the ability to store up calories as fat was an advantage. Because this trait increased the chances of survival during famine, more and more humans passed it on to the next generation. Biologists call this explanation for why we get fat the "thrifty-gene hypothesis."

Did the tendency to store excess fat predispose our ancestors to diabetes and heart disease? Undoubtedly, it did, but their dietary and activity patterns protected them from these conditions.

How Insulin Resistance Affects Your Health

Excessive demands for insulin and wide fluctuations of blood glucose levels, which are typical of unchecked insulin resistance, cause myriad health problems, including the following:

- **Type 2 diabetes:** If insulin production can't keep up with demand, glucose levels begin to rise, causing type 2, or adult-onset, diabetes. Uncontrolled diabetes literally sugar-coats tissues and can eventually lead to eye, kidney, and blood vessel damage.
- **Beta cell burnout:** The beta cells of the pancreas, which secrete insulin, also make a substance called *amylin*. When they secrete excessive amounts of insulin, they also produce excessive amounts of amylin. High concentrations of amylin turn into an insoluble sludge called amyloid that damages the very cells that secrete it. Biopsies of the pancreases of

patients with type 2 diabetes often show replacement of insulin-secreting cells by amyloid.

- **Hypoglycemia (low blood sugar):** One of the earliest signs of insulin resistance is what's commonly called low blood sugar. It might seem strange that a condition that leads to high blood sugar could cause low blood sugar, but when insulin-resistant individuals go 3 or 4 hours without eating, they often experience weakness, poor concentration, and a strong craving for food, all of which are promptly relieved by eating. Actually, the term *low blood sugar* is a misnomer. When the pancreas has to make large amounts of insulin, it often overshoots, causing glucose levels to fall too fast. This triggers a surge of another hormone, adrenaline, which stops glucose from falling. It's the adrenaline—not low blood glucose—that causes the shakiness and poor concentration typical of hypoglycemia. Adrenaline highs and lows typically occur several times a day, causing quirky eating patterns, frayed nerves, and end-of-the-day fatigue.
- **Heart and blood vessel disease:** When your body gets more glucose than it can handle, your liver turns the excess to fat globules, which travel through your bloodstream to your fat deposits in the form of triglyceride. Although triglyceride doesn't damage arteries directly, high concentrations reduce blood levels of "good cholesterol," HDL, which raises the risk of blood vessel disease even when bad cholesterol levels are normal. (I talk about this more in Chapter 11.)
- **Menstrual difficulties:** In women, insulin resistance sometimes brings on polycystic ovary syndrome (PCOS), which causes irregular periods, ovarian cysts, abnormal hair growth, and acne. PCOS is the leading cause of female infertility in the United States, affecting approximately 6 percent of women. It can be treated with a low-starch diet, exercise, and insulin-sensitizing medication.
- **Sleep apnea:** Accumulation of fat in the abdomen and neck typical of insulin resistance interferes with breathing during sleep. This causes excessive snoring and aggravates sleep apnea, a form of erratic breathing that robs sleep of its restfulness.

How to Tell If You Are Insulin Resistant

Although doctors recognized that many of their patients had insulin resistance, they had no idea how common it was until researchers tested large segments of the population. According to a recent government study, 22 percent of the American population has insulin resistance—44 percent of those more than 50 years old. Among individuals who are 30 pounds overweight or more, the incidence is 85 percent. The bottom line is this: If you're overweight, you probably have insulin resistance.

Measuring insulin resistance directly is a tedious laboratory procedure usually done only in research centers. However, doctors found that they could accurately surmise its presence by looking for signs of the metabolic syndrome. Here are the criteria, defined by the National Cholesterol Education Program, for diagnosing it. If you have any three of the following five characteristics, you probably have insulin resistance.

1. *A tendency to accumulate fat in the abdomen:* abdominal girth measured at your navel of 38 inches or more if you're a male or 34 inches if you're a female, or a waist measurement more than 95 percent of your hip circumference measured around your buttocks if you're a male, 85 percent if you're a female
2. *High blood triglyceride level:* a triglyceride level greater than 150
3. *Low blood level of good cholesterol:* an HDL level below 40 if you are male or 50 if you are female
4. *Borderline or high blood pressure:* systolic blood pressure greater than 130 or diastolic blood pressure greater than 85
5. *Borderline or high blood glucose:* fasting blood glucose level greater than 110

Super Xers

Viewing him from behind, you could hardly tell Henry was overweight. He had narrow hips and not much fat on his arms or legs. However, in profile you could see that he had a potbelly. His abdomen extended several inches beyond his belt. His girth was 42 inches. His triglyceride level was 280.

When Henry reduced his intake of refined carbohydrates and started walking regularly, he lost weight. Impressed at how easy it was, he began testing himself to see how much rich food he could get away with eating. He was amazed to find that he could consume generous amounts of fat and protein—even more than he was naturally inclined to eat—yet continue to lose weight.

I often encounter patients who have especially flagrant signs of syndrome X—abdominal girth more than 42 inches for males or 38 inches for females and triglyceride levels greater than 225. I call such folks Super Xers. It's gratifying to work with these individuals, because they usually respond dramatically to measures that relieve insulin resistance.

For Super Xers, eliminating carbohydrates is like taking away a toxin from people who have been poisoning themselves. As long as they avoid refined carbohydrates, they seem to be immune to gaining weight.

How You Can Reverse Insulin Resistance

The good news is that if you have insulin resistance, you don't have to put up with it. Few conditions in medicine are such a cinch to treat. It's easy to stop the blood glucose surges that trigger excessive insulin secretion and restore your slow-twitch muscles' sensitivity to insulin. You can do it by cutting out just a handful of bland, unexciting foods and engaging in some physical activity that even couch potatoes don't mind doing. If you do both of those things, your insulin levels will drop like a rock, your metabolism will fall back into balance, and probably, without trying to cut calories or engaging in strenuous exercise, you will steadily lose weight.

Is this hard to do? Put it this way: You won't find an easier way to lose weight. Later in the book, you will learn that if you remove starch from your diet, you won't have to worry much about sugar, and it turns out that starch is essentially tasteless. In your mouth a small fraction of it breaks down into glucose, which you can taste, but most of it ends up in your stomach without your tasting it. Thus, when you eliminate starch, you mainly just remove

IN THEIR OWN WORDS

Name and Age: Xan, 43

Pounds Lost: 25 in 5 months

Health Benefits: Decreased blood pressure to 100/55, dropped triglycerides from 142 to 96, increased HDL cholesterol, dropped A1C (a diabetes marker) from 5.7 to 5.4, dropped two pants sizes

"Someone asked me after the first 2 weeks if I'd had 'some work' done!"

Despite significant "dietary discipline" (about 1,500 calories per day) and regular exercise for more than 5 years, I was putting on about 10 pounds per year for the past 4 years and was feeling completely out of control. I had tried Atkins a decade ago, but found it completely unsustainable. I knew I needed a new approach, and I suspected that my problem was related to the endocrine system. So I found your program and adopted your recommendations with the same spirit you seem to have given them—with moderation and an eye toward the long term.

flavorless paste. Most of the satisfying flavors and textures in your regular diet stay.

Another reason it's easy to eliminate starch is that it contains no essential vitamins or minerals. This is important because even the slightest shortage of vital nutrients creates food cravings. But because there is no biological need for starch, getting rid of it creates no deficiencies. Indeed, no creature ever suffered poor health for lack of starch.

As for activating your slow-twitch muscle fibers, if you ascribe to the no-pain, no-gain philosophy of exercise, you might find what I'm going to tell you hard to believe, but there are muscles in your body that require virtually no effort to exercise. A good

In just 5 months. I have lost 25 pounds, my A1C has dropped from 5.7 to 5.4, my total cholesterol has stayed about the same (around 215) but the HDL has increased, my triglycerides have dropped from 142 to 96, and my blood pressure, though not high in recent years, was down to 100/55 last week.

Besides those important numbers, I have dropped two pants sizes, and the puffiness is gone from my hands and face. (I actually had someone ask me after the first 2 weeks if I'd had "some work" done!) And on Thanksgiving Day, I plan on running my first 5-K. I had been running for about 5 months before I changed my diet, and while it had its benefits, it was not nearly as enjoyable as it is now. I am 43 years old and feel better than I have in 15 years.

Another benefit for someone who is a bit of a "food snob" like myself is that I am eating normal food. And I am eating more than I did before (by an average of about 500 calories per day), so I am not walking around hungry all the time. To be truthful, I am never hungry.

I now know how to eat, exercise, and live in a way that makes me both healthy and happy. I finally feel like I have some control.

example is your diaphragm, the main breathing muscle beneath your rib cage. How much effort does it take to breathe? The reason your diaphragm can work effortlessly without your even thinking about it is that it is powered by slow-twitch muscle fibers, which, as it turns out, are the ones that determine your body's sensitivity to insulin. In other words, the muscles you need to exercise to relieve insulin resistance are precisely the ones that require the least effort to use. Even folks who dislike exercise can do it and actually enjoy it. (I cover this in more detail in Chapter 8.)

The combination of removing starch from your diet and activating your slow-twitch muscle fibers is certainly the least complicated way to lose weight. Although I have included many delicious low-starch recipes in this book, there really is no need for special food preparation. You can go to the same restaurants as before, eat alongside everybody else, and attract no attention. You only need to avoid a handful of foods, which you can quickly learn to recognize.

Start Today

Don't wait any longer to get started. At your next meal, hold off eating any bread, potatoes, or rice until you finish everything else, and then, if you must, have about a quarter of the amount of these foods that you usually eat. *Remember, don't deprive yourself of food.* Make up for eating less starch by helping yourself to more of everything else. This is not a calorie-cutting diet. It's a way of reducing the amount of insulin your body has to make.

If, in addition to reducing your intake of those three foods, you walk 30 minutes every other day, after a few days your body chemistry will function much differently than it did before. Your beta cells will have to make only a fraction of the insulin they were producing previously, your blood sugar will stop fluctuating wildly, and fat globules will disappear from your blood. You will have removed the driving force behind your weight gain.

You might also notice that you feel better. Highs and lows of blood glucose cause your body to make excessive amounts of adrenaline, which jars your nerves and leaves you feeling burned out and exhausted. Smoothing out these fluctuations makes you feel calmer and gives you more energy later in the day.

Believing in What You're Doing and Knowing How to Do It

It is possible to lose weight by either eliminating foods that require a lot of insulin or exercising to increase your muscles' sensitivity to insulin, but the secret is to do both. The two approaches potentiate one another—that is, one makes the other more effective. Eliminating blood glucose surges improves your muscles' sensitivity to insulin, and improving your muscles' sensitivity to insulin stabilizes your blood glucose levels.

Although the changes you need to make to relieve insulin resistance are as small as they can possibly be and still produce weight loss, they are changes nonetheless, and they need to be permanent. This is not a fad diet meant to be started and stopped when you have reached a goal. To ingrain new eating habits and activity patterns, you need to believe in what you're doing and know how to do it.

In the next few chapters, I'm going to show you the science behind the principles I have outlined here. Once you understand what made you gain weight, you'll see clearly what you need to do. You'll learn what the easiest, most effective way is to stop your body from overproducing insulin. If instead of trying to starve yourself you concentrate on correcting what caused you to gain weight, you'll be astonished at how easy it is to shed pounds and keep them off for good.

2

Starch Toxicity: How Staples Turned Out to Be Toxins

O ne thing is for sure: If your weight has been creeping up lately, you're not alone. A lot of us have the same problem. How did so many of us get this way?

To gain weight, you have to take in more calories than you burn off. Otherwise, your body would defy the laws of thermodynamics. The question is not whether you consumed more calories than you burned off but *why* you consumed more calories than you burned off. Your body has weight-regulating mechanisms that are supposed to balance food intake with energy expenditure. What's throwing those systems out of kilter?

You hear a lot these days about toxins in the food chain—things like mercury, PCBs, and iodine. The alleged culprit is usually a chemical introduced into the environment by humans and found to be harmful to laboratory animals when ingested in large doses. The media sound the alarm, people fuss about it for a while, and then the hysteria dies down. No one seems to get sick from these things. As a doctor, I've personally never seen any illness I could relate to mercury, PCB, or iodine toxicity. It makes interesting news, but the amounts of these pollutants in our food are usually much too small to make us sick.

However, every day I see patients suffering from the effects of another toxin. It's a mixture of two chemicals, *amylase* and *amylopectin,* that people introduced into their food only recently in the span of human existence. But unlike the toxins you hear about in the news, this one exists in our food in, frankly, toxic concentrations. Although its effects are subtle, sometimes taking years to do their damage, it often leads to progressive disability, disease, and death. Where are we getting this toxin? We make a point of adding it to nearly every meal we eat. It's the main ingredient of bread, potatoes, and rice and is more commonly known as *starch*.

Bread, Potatoes, and Rice: How "Natural" Are They?

Starch is, in fact, the same tasteless paste laundries use for stiffening shirt collars. The word *starch* comes from the Middle English word *sterchen,* "to stiffen," which, as it turns out, is what it does to your arteries. However, most of us don't think of starch as a toxin, because the foods that contain it are so familiar to us. We've been eating bread, potatoes, and rice all our lives, as have our parents and grandparents. Actually, many people can get away with eating large amounts of starch without harmful effects because they either are genetically resistant to its harmful effects or have certain activity patterns that protect them. However, for those of us who are susceptible—which includes about 40 percent of the population—starch toxicity is a menacing reality. Consumption of amounts common in our modern diet can lead to serious medical problems like diabetes and heart disease—but usually not before causing years of unsightly, frustrating obesity.

When you're a kid, your body can handle a lot of starch. Your pancreas makes plenty of insulin, and your tissues respond very well to it. However, when you grow up—especially if you have a genetic predisposition to insulin resistance—the way your body metabolizes glucose changes. Your pancreas continues to make plenty of insulin, but your body begins losing its responsiveness to it. As a result, your pancreas has to make increasing amounts of insulin to keep your blood glucose levels down. As time passes, your body's ability to produce insulin begins to lag. If the pancreas can't secrete enough insulin to overcome insulin resistance, glucose starts backing up in the bloodstream, the condition we call type 2 or adult-onset diabetes.

The tissues that line blood vessels are particularly vulnerable to high blood glucose levels. Diabetes eventually leads to blood-vessel disease, the most common cause of death and disability in the industrialized world. However, diabetes is only the late stage of starch toxicity. Profound body chemistry disturbances precede diabetes by decades, causing quirky appetite regulation and imbalances between good and bad cholesterol that promote cholesterol buildup in arteries. The most frustrating problem starch toxicity causes, though, is a tendency to accumulate excess body fat.

Starch Poisoning: The Price of Civilization

How did the foods we rely on most to prevent hunger—so-called staples like wheat, potatoes, and rice—end up causing so much trouble? For millions of years, our prehistoric ancestors roamed the earth, hunting game and gathering natural vegetation for food. Starch was a minuscule part of their diet. They consumed it only in tiny quantities locked in the protective husks of seeds that were not particularly appealing to eat.

In nature, starch provides a concentrated source of energy for seeds to sprout. The seeds of grasses native to regions with long, hot dry seasons and short, temperate wet seasons are especially high in starch, which serves to jump-start these plants so they can mature quickly during short growing seasons. Impermeable husks protect the seeds from the sun and predators during the dry season.

Around 10,000 years ago—very recently in the span of human existence—people living in the eastern Mediterranean region and South Asia, where wheat and rice grew naturally, figured out how to extract the starchy cores of the seeds of these grasses from their protective husks by grinding them between rocks and letting the wind blow away the chaff. They learned to use these grains to stave off starvation when meat and fresh vegetation were scarce. For the first time, humans discovered a plentiful source of calories for which they didn't have to compete with other predators and that they could store for months.

Later our ancestors found that by adding water and heating the starchy filling—the "flour"—of these kernels, they could make them more palatable. As time passed, they discovered more ways to make wheat taste better. They added fat to flour to make it moist, leavened it with yeast to lighten it, and added sugar to sweeten it. The cultivation of wheat in the West, rice in Asia, and corn in the New World was a boon to humankind. These staples provided—and continue to provide—an efficient means of feeding people. Because they all have to be processed or "refined" before they can be eaten— they are inedible in their natural form—they have come to be called *refined carbohydrates*. Of all the foods humans eat, refined carbohydrates supply by far the most calories with the least investment of land, labor, and capital.

Not only did the domestication of wheat, rice, and corn change the human diet, but it also transformed civilization. The ability to stockpile food supplies freed humans from having to forage constantly. This encouraged cooperation, division of labor, and eventually formation of governmental structures. Along with government and spare manpower came armies of conquest. Eventually, the eastern Mediterranean and South Asian regions gave rise to the dominant civilizations of the world, and reliance on starchy staples spread to most societies on Earth.

A Monumental Change in Body Chemistry

The cultivation of refined carbohydrates represented a major change in the human body's chemical environment. Prehistoric humans ate only small amounts of starch entangled in fiber and encapsulated in impervious husks. It took hours for their digestive tracts to process such foods. It was a shock to the human metabolism when, instead of the occasional granule of starch, people began consuming cupfuls at every meal in concentrated, rapidly digestible form.

Your body handles refined carbohydrates differently from any other kind of food. As soon as starch hits your stomach, it breaks down to glucose, which short-circuits the digestive process, going directly into your bloodstream without traveling more than a few inches down your intestinal tract. Within minutes, your blood glucose levels shoot up to heights never experienced by your prehistoric ancestors.

If genetic changes are needed to handle this sudden and recent change in digestive physiology, the human race has not had enough time to evolve them. Genetic adaptation requires hundreds of thousands of years, but starchy staples have been around for only about 10,000—a mere tick of the evolutionary clock. It isn't surprising that the shift to refined carbohydrates that has occurred in the last few thousand years has had a profound effect on human health.

The Two Faces of Starch Toxicity

Worldwide, excessive starch consumption manifests itself in two ways, depending on whether there is sufficient intake of other foods. In underdeveloped countries where populations rely heavily on starchy staples for survival, refined flour, rice, and potatoes have supplanted other sources of nutrition, many of which are vital to good health. Because starch provides little in the way of vitamins, minerals, or protein, deficiencies of these nutrients are rampant in these areas. In parts of Africa and Asia that rely heavily on starchy staples, as much as 40 percent of the population suffers from iron-poor blood caused by lack of meat and iron-containing vegetables. Iron deficiency is so widespread in some countries that it measurably affects their economies. Another major health problem in poor countries is kwashiorkor, a disease of protein deficiency. This condition weakens the immune system and causes children to die of otherwise minor illnesses like measles and chickenpox. Many children in these regions suffer from rickets, a disease of calcium deficiency that causes weakening and bending of bones. These conditions are practically unheard of in areas with adequate supplies of meat and dairy products.

Excessive consumption of refined carbohydrates causes a different set of problems in wealthier countries. In these parts of the world, people can choose from a wide variety of foods, so vitamin, mineral, and protein deficiencies are rare. But while folks in developed countries aren't dependent on starch for survival, they still eat large amounts of it. The problem is not lack of more nutritious foods by starch but rather the toxic effects of starch itself. Excessive amounts of refined carbohydrates are causing epidemics of obesity and diabetes.

Why Do We Eat So Much Starch?

Economics drive our dependence on starch. In the first place, bread, potatoes, and rice are cheap. People can eat their fill without spending a lot of money. Not only is starch affordable for consumers, it's a cheap ingredient for packaged food manufacturers. Best of all, companies can obtain patents on their processing techniques so other firms can't compete with them. This allows them to sell their products at high profit margins.

The potential for large profits encourages companies to think up ever more imaginative ways to prepare and market starch. High profit margins allow for more revenue to be spent on advertising. Consequently, firms that manufacture brand-name processed foods, such as crackers, chips, and breakfast cereals, advertise heavily. Unlike producers of fresh produce who can't obtain patents on their products. Without the ability to exclude competition, suppliers of fresh fruit, vegetables, meat, and dairy products have to maintain competitive prices. Because their profit margins are so slim, the only way they can make a profit is by keeping their overhead down. Consequently, they can't afford to advertise much. You rarely see television ads for fresh produce.

As a rule, when others are paying for the ingredients of the food you eat, their economic incentive is to feed you starch. That's why restaurants are happy to see you fill up on bread, potatoes, and rice. The profit margin on a McDonald's hamburger is razor thin. Fast-food restaurants make most of their money selling french fries and soft drinks.

The Obesity Epidemic: How America Got Fat

In 1962, 13 percent of the American population was obese (defined as being 30 pounds or more overweight), and that percentage had remained stable for decades. Then, around 1970, the numbers suddenly started rising. By 1998, the proportion of obese Americans more than doubled to 31 percent, and the incidence of diabetes, which is often brought on by excessive weight gain, rose sixfold. What caused the obesity rate to suddenly shoot up like this?

You'll hear many explanations for why so many people are overweight these days. Proponents of various theories usually cite some evidence to support their opinions, but the data are often flawed. It's hard to study people's diets. You can't put humans in pens and control what they eat the way you can with laboratory animals. In a sense, though, we all live in a sort of pen—the one defined by our national borders. As it turns out, the US Department of Agriculture keeps close tabs on the types of foods Americans eat, and the National Health and Nutrition Examination Survey carefully tracks people's heights and weights. If you combine these two sources of data, you can gain some compelling insights as to why we are gaining weight.

In the 1950s and 1960s, Americans reveled in their ability to eat fresh farm food, including eggs, meat, and dairy products. For the first time in history, modernized agricultural techniques, refrigeration, and rapid transportation made these goods available and affordable for most citizens. Americans remembered harder times during the Great Depression, when people suffered from iron-deficiency anemia and rickets caused by lack of adequate nutrition. To be able to enjoy fresh produce, which prevented such conditions, was a privilege.

Then, around 1970, something came along that chilled America's ardor for eggs, meat, and dairy products. Government agencies and medical organizations, concerned about the rising incidence of heart disease, started recommending low-fat, low-cholesterol diets—not just for people prone to artery disease but for everybody. The theory, later proven wrong, was that reducing the cholesterol in food would reduce the cholesterol in people's blood and prevent heart attacks. This public health effort coincided with a rise in popularity of vegetarianism and a period of rampant inflation of prices for fresh produce, meat, and dairy products. The result was an abrupt shift in eating patterns away from eggs, red

Table 2.1 Annual Consumption of Red Meat, Eggs, and Milk, 1970 versus 1997

	Consumption per Person		
Type of Food	1970	1997	Change 1970 to 1997
Red meat	132 lb	111 lb	Down 16%
Eggs	309 eggs	239 eggs	Down 23%
Milk fat (equivalent in whole milk)	114 qt	55 qt	Down 52%

Source: US Department of Agriculture National Nutrient Database

meat, and dairy food. Table 2.1 shows how consumption of these foods has changed since 1970. Clearly, Americans did exactly what government agencies and doctors told them to do: They cut down on fat- and cholesterol-containing foods. We are now eating 16 percent less red meat, 23 percent fewer eggs, and 52 percent less milk fat per person than we did 40 years ago.

If you eat less of one kind of food, you're bound to eat more of another. Indeed, Americans are now eating more carbohydrates—plant-based foods—but not the healthy kind, like fresh fruits and vegetables. The biggest change in the American diet in the last 40 years has been a dramatic increase in consumption of *refined* carbohydrates: flour products, rice, and potatoes. As you can see from Table 2.2, we are eating 48 percent more flour, 186 percent more rice, and 131 percent more frozen potatoes, mainly in the form of french fries, than we did in 1970.

Table 2.2 Annual Consumption of Flour, Rice, and Potatoes, 1970 versus 1997

	Consumption per Person		
Type of Food	1970	1997	Change 1970 to 1997
Flour	135 lb	200 lb	Up 48%
Rice	7 lb	20 lb	Up 186%
Frozen potato products (mainly french fries)	13 lb	30 lb	Up 131%

Source: US Department of Agriculture National Nutrient Database

The Wheat-Obesity Link

America's largest source of starch by far is wheat. The graph in Figure 2.1 compares the average wheat consumption per person over the last 40 years with the percentage of the population that is 30 pounds or more overweight. You can see that as soon as wheat consumption started rising in the 1970s, the obesity rate did the same. The message is clear: The more wheat Americans eat, the fatter they get.

Figure 2.1 Obesity Rate versus Annual Wheat Consumption per Person (1961–2000)

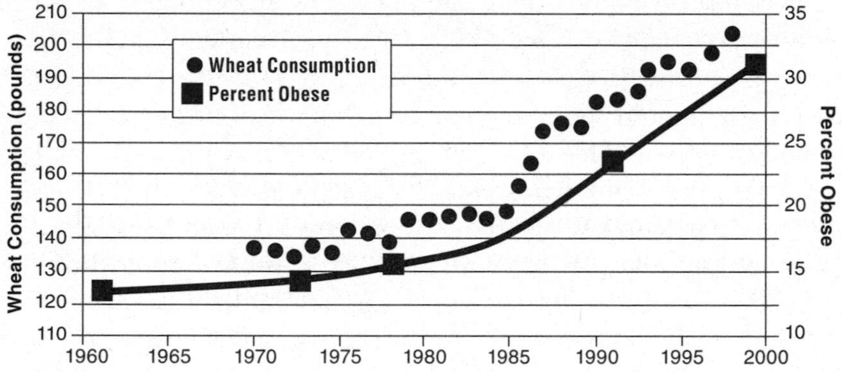

Source: National Center for Health Statistics Third National Health and Nutrition Examination Survey and US Department of Agriculture National Nutrient Database

What about Sugar?

Another carbohydrate we are eating more of is sugar. We Americans are consuming 26 percent more sugar per person than we did before 1970. But we're not eating it in the form of candy. Candy consumption has actually remained stable over the past 40 years. We are consuming more sugar because adults are eating it in flour products such as rolls, doughnuts, cookies, and cakes, and kids are consuming it in soft drinks.

Because the starch in flour is essentially flavorless, you need to doctor it up to make it taste good. On the other hand, sugar is overwhelmingly sweet; you have to dilute it to make it palatable. However, if you combine starch with sugar, you give it some flavor and you tone down the sweetness of the sugar. One reason adults are consuming more sugar is because they're eating more sweetened starches such as cookies, cakes, and pastries.

What about so-called high-fructose corn syrup? Researchers have pointed out that we started getting fatter around the time we began consuming more of it. Some nutritionists think that fructose might be more fattening than regular cane sugar. However, there's another explanation. In the 1970s, the US government stopped paying farmers to limit corn production as a way of propping up prices, and started encouraging them to grow more. This created a huge oversupply of corn. Producers had to come up with a way to sell more corn products, so they did what your digestive tract does to corn: They turned it into sugar. They started selling corn syrup as a cheap replacement for cane sugar.

No doubt, the large-scale replacement of cane sugar by corn syrup contributed to obesity and diabetes, but not because it's chemically much different from regular sugar. Cane sugar is 50 percent fructose; high-fructose corn syrup is 55 percent fructose. Indeed, the main reason corn syrup has made America's diabetes and obesity problems worse is that *it's so cheap.* Now kids can afford to buy soda in 20-ounce bottles instead of 7-ounce ones—the way it was sold before cheap corn syrup became available.

The Big "Fat" Lie

What about our supposed nemesis, fat? Government agencies, medical organizations, and vegetarian groups tried to convince us for years that we were gaining weight because we were eating too much fat, but that notion is so far off base you wonder if someone was putting us on. The truth is, we're eating considerably *less* fat and cholesterol than we did before the obesity epidemic began. Indeed, researchers have found that as people gain weight, they eat less fat and more carbohydrates. Clearly, dietary fat is not what's causing our weight problems.

IN THEIR OWN WORDS

Name and Age: Betsy, 56

Pounds Lost: 50 in 10 months

Health Benefits: Increased energy, reduced joint pain, lost four dress sizes

"It's not even a diet!"

I had tried all kinds of different diets in my life, and had pretty much given up on the idea of losing weight. I tried several, including liquid fasts and several low-calorie diets. I always gained the weight back quickly. I told a friend that I wished I could lose weight for a reunion. She suggested I follow Dr. Thompson's program.

I did what the book said. I reduced my glycemic load and started walking a couple of miles a day, and was flabbergasted at the results. I lost 50 pounds in 10 months.

What amazes me is how easy it is. It's not even a diet! It's just a different way of eating (and exercising). At restaurants, I eat more salad, beef, and chicken and push away the starchy things.

During some of the other diets, I felt weak and dizzy. With this one, I felt better than ever: My energy improved, my joints stopped aching. I no longer felt helpless about my weight.

Even though fast-food restaurants provide, on average, only 12 percent of America's caloric intake, they are frequently blamed for making folks fat. The reason given is that these places serve up too much "fatty" food. But the next time you see a supersize meal in McDonald's or Burger King, ask yourself how much of what you are looking at is meat and dairy product and how much is bun, french fries, and soft drink—that is, how much is fat, and how much is starch and sugar? Fast food isn't so much fatty as it is starchy and sugary.

Too Much Starch, Not Enough Exercise, or Both?

As a child, I remember visiting my grandparents, who were dairy farmers. My grandmother baked huge trays of cinnamon rolls every week. She kept her pantry stocked with fresh homemade bread. She boiled big pots of potatoes and served them mashed for dinner and fried for breakfast. Her icebox was filled with eggs, meat, and dairy products at all times. Her family could eat as much rich food as they wanted whenever they wanted. Talk about convenience foods—they didn't even have to drive to a fast-food restaurant. Why didn't they get fat?

Clearly, there's more to our obesity problems than the food we eat, be it starchy or fatty. The other side of the weight gain equation is the lack of physical activity that characterizes our modern lifestyle. My grandparents and their children didn't get fat because they did several hours of physical work every day. Indeed, researchers who study the effects of lifestyle on obesity find a much closer correlation with physical activity than with eating patterns.

Statistics show that the more time people spend commuting to work in automobiles, the more likely they are to be overweight. A while back, I saw a photograph in the *Seattle Times* taken in 1915 of a group of businessmen in downtown Seattle, and it struck me that they were all slim. I wondered what they did differently from us modern folks. They were wearing business suits, so I doubted they did physical work all day. The only difference I could think of from the businesspeople of today was that they probably walked to work; in those days, most Seattleites lived a mile or two from downtown. Not long afterward, I gave up my downtown parking place, left my car at home, and started walking to work. That was 5 years ago, and I still walk to work. I have been surprised at how much I enjoy it.

Exercise does more than just burn off calories while you are doing it. It revs up your metabolism, activates hormonal systems, and increases your body's sensitivity to insulin for days afterward.

When you exercise, you literally burn more calories while you sleep. Scientists have found that the higher the level of physical activity, the more precisely the body's weight-regulating mechanisms work. In other words, when you exercise, your body more accurately matches the calories you take in with the energy you burn off.

Nevertheless, although lack of exercise set the stage for Americans to gain weight, it doesn't explain why the obesity rate suddenly started rising 30 years ago. Activity levels had been declining for years. In fact, the largest reductions occurred in the first half of the 20th century, when Americans stopped doing farmwork and started driving cars, but before 1970 the obesity rate was half of what it is now and had remained stable for decades.

It's true that if we did as much physical work and walked as much as our ancestors did, there would probably be no obesity epidemic, but what has changed the most in the past four decades has not been our exercise habits. It's been our diet. We're eating less fat but much more starch. The skyrocketing obesity rate of the last 40 years correlates precisely with a dramatic increase in our consumption of refined carbohydrates.

Actually, starch toxicity isn't so different from other epidemics that have decimated human populations over the centuries, and it isn't the only disease to be wrongly blamed on character shortcomings. People used to think that leprosy and tuberculosis were caused by lack of moral fiber. Humans conquered the scourges of the past only when they abandoned the notion that character defects caused them and began looking for physiological causes. The obesity epidemic will be halted only when we stop focusing on personal shortcomings and begin addressing the metabolic disturbances that cause weight problems, including our biologically unnatural dependence on refined carbohydrates.

3

What Makes Bad Carbs Bad

He wasn't the first to discover it, but he was probably the most persistent. In the 1960s, New York cardiologist Dr. Robert C. Atkins found that when his overweight patients cut out plant-based foods—fruits, vegetables, grains, and sugar—many of them lost weight, even while eating generous amounts of rich, fatty foods. Remarkably, they seemed to be able to shed pounds without trying to cut calories.

Encouraged by these observations, Atkins devised for his patients a weight-loss diet that eliminated all carbohydrates. The only ones he allowed were green leafy vegetables in limited quantities. The results were impressive. Many of his patients experienced dramatic weight loss even while consuming large amounts of foods strictly forbidden by other diets, including liberal amounts of meat, cheese, and butter. In his book *Dr. Atkins' Diet Revolution*, published in 1971, dieters found a way to lose weight while continuing to eat many of their favorite foods—again, without trying to cut calories.

Unfortunately, Atkins's timing couldn't have been worse. Researchers had recently discovered links between high blood cholesterol and heart disease. In those days, nutritionists took the adage "You are what you eat" literally. They thought people had high blood cholesterol simply because they ate too much cholesterol, and got fat simply because they ate too much fat. Because most of the cholesterol and fat in the American diet came from animal products, they figured the best way to lower cholesterol and lose weight was to cut out eggs, red meat, and dairy products. This advice also resonated with people's vegetarian and animal rights beliefs. Not only was such a diet better for you, it was kinder to animals. A low-fat, low-cholesterol diet high in carbohydrates seemed to be the way to go.

Atkins's conflicting recommendations to eat fewer carbohydrates and *more* meat and dairy products soon became heresy. He was actually called before a congressional committee to defend his views and was publicly derided. It seemed for a while that his detractors had won. At the urging of the government and the medical community, and despite lack of proof of effectiveness, America started moving toward a lower-fat, lower-cholesterol, *higher*carbohydrate diet.

The Weight-Loss Power of Low-Carb Eating

Atkins was an experienced heart specialist. He knew that the old saying "You are what you eat" is misleading. When it comes to fat and cholesterol, you really aren't what you eat. Your body can quickly transform carbohydrates to fat and cholesterol. In fact, unlike fat and cholesterol, carbohydrates cause your pancreas to secrete insulin, a hormone notorious for causing weight gain.

Atkins also knew that reducing dietary cholesterol didn't lower blood cholesterol much. Your body makes its own cholesterol— about three times as much as you eat. If you reduce the amount of cholesterol in your diet, your liver just makes more. If you eat more, your liver makes less. The level of cholesterol in your blood is determined not by how much cholesterol you eat but by how efficient your system is at getting rid of it, and that's mainly a matter of genetics. When it comes to cholesterol, who your parents are is much more important than what you eat.

The more experience Atkins gained, the more certain he became that a low-carb, liberalized-fat diet was safe for most people and more effective for losing weight than low-fat diets. In 1991, more than 20 years after his first book, he published *Dr. Atkins' New*

Diet Revolution. The enormous impact this book made was as much a matter of timing as it was content. Twenty years of low-fat, low-cholesterol advice seemed only to have made Americans fatter. People were desperate to lose weight and ready to try anything: diet pills, jaw wiring, stomach surgery—whatever did the job. Finally, some folks started ignoring concerns about cholesterol and returning to the Atkins diet. They again discovered that it worked. People who had failed to lose weight with other programs often succeeded with the Atkins diet. They told their friends, and, for the second time, Atkins's strict low-carb, high-fat diet became popular.

The resurrection of the Atkins diet in the 1990s was a grass-roots movement. The medical community had nothing to do with it. For the most part, doctors and nutritionists were chagrined. Mired in low-fat, low-cholesterol orthodoxy, they feared an epidemic of high blood cholesterol, but the scourge never materialized. One difference between the 1970s and the 1990s was that in the nineties, doctors routinely checked cholesterol levels and were better able to detect heart disease. As it turns out, they didn't find any tendency for low-carb diets to cause heart problems or even raise cholesterol. When their patients lost weight, they just seemed healthier for it.

In the late 1990s, researchers finally put the low-carb, liberalized-fat diet to the test, comparing it head-to-head with traditional low-fat, calorie-restricted diets. They found that Atkins was right after all: Low-carb diets were more effective than low-fat diets. People lost more weight, and, in most cases, their blood cholesterol levels improved. Best of all, they didn't have to go hungry. They could eat until they were satisfied and still shed pounds.

Atkins was vindicated. Sadly, he died in an accident a month before the nation's most reputable medical journal, the *New England Journal of Medicine,* published the results of those studies.

By this time, study after study had failed to show that low-cholesterol, low-fat diets prevented heart disease or even lowered blood cholesterol levels much. Then, in 2006, researchers released the results of the Women's Health Initiative Dietary Modification Trial, an enormous, government-sponsored study designed to settle the question of whether low-cholesterol, low-fat diets lowered cholesterol or prevented heart disease. Researchers randomly assigned 48,835 women to either of two groups. One group received intensive low-fat, low-cholesterol dietary counseling by certified nutritionists. The other group received no training. The 19,541 women who got the counseling attended 18 low-cholesterol, low-fat diet training sessions the first year and one session every 3 months thereafter for 8 years.

Follow-up interviews confirmed that the group of women who received the training succeeded in lowering their fat and cholesterol intake, but it did no good. After 8 years, their average cholesterol levels fell less than 2 percent—not nearly enough to affect their risk of heart disease—and there was no difference whatsoever in their heart attack or stroke rates.

Does diet affect cholesterol? You bet it does, but not the way you think. Your risk of heart disease depends as much on your blood levels of HDL, or "good cholesterol," as it does on your bad cholesterol levels. HDL actually removes cholesterol from your arteries. As it turns out, you can raise your levels of good cholesterol, not by eliminating dietary fat and cholesterol, *but by reducing carbs.*

This is especially true if you add some exercise. In the early 2000s, researchers released the results of several studies showing that low-carb, liberalized-fat diets raise HDL modestly, about 5 percent, and for years, it has been known that regular exercise raises HDL levels modestly, also about 5 percent. However, if you do both—cut carbs *and* exercise—you can quadruple the benefits. In 2010, the *Annals of Internal Medicine* published the results of a study showing that a low-carb, liberalized-fat diet combined with 50 minutes of walking 5 days a week raised HDL levels on average 23 percent—as much as any medication available today.

Strict Low-Carb Diets: Powerful but Not Sustainable

If you're overweight and do what Atkins recommended—cut out virtually all carbohydrates except leafy green vegetables—you'll see dramatic things happen. You'll lose weight while consuming an amazingly rich diet. The level of fat in your blood (triglyceride) will plummet, your blood glucose levels will fall, and your good cholesterol levels will rise. If you're typical, your bad cholesterol levels won't change much or will fall slightly.

People who try the Atkins diet are often astonished at how fast the pounds melt away. I've seen patients lose weight so fast they thought something was wrong with them. Although I don't advocate such rapid weight loss, when I see such dramatic responses, it's apparent to me that there's more to cutting carbs than reducing calories. It's as if people who have been inadvertently poisoning themselves for years discover the toxin and stop ingesting it.

What's remarkable about cutting carbs is not just that you lose weight but that you do it without "dieting"—without consciously trying to reduce the amount of food you eat. When your body stops overproducing insulin, you lose weight naturally. You don't have to count calories. You can eat until you're satisfied and still shed pounds. Carbohydrate restriction is indeed a powerful weapon for losing weight.

Nevertheless, while it might be easier to shed pounds with a low-carb diet than with a low-fat approach, most folks who go on the Atkins diet don't stick with it for long. Although you would think that a diet that allows you to eat all the rich food you want would be easy to stick with, as it turns out, most people who go on the Atkins diet eventually go back to their old ways. The problem is *food cravings*. Fruits and vegetables are full of vitamins, minerals, and fiber that are essential to good health. When you try to remove those nutrients from your diet, your body fights back, and you begin craving the missing foods. If you have a sweet tooth, you also miss sweets, not necessarily to satisfy hunger, but just for the pleasure of tasting them. Eventually, your cravings for the forbidden foods overcome your motivation to continue, and you go back to your old ways. The reality is that the choice of foods allowed by the Atkins diet, and its more recent counterpart, the South Beach diet, is just too narrow for most people to tolerate for long.

The Atkins craze eventually died down. But just as the public was losing interest in strict low-carb diets, nutritional scientists were discovering ways that people could benefit from the weight-loss power of carbohydrate restriction without the diet-wrecking narrowness of these diets. To understand how you can enjoy satisfying amounts of a much wider variety of foods and still lose weight, you need to know the differences between good carbs and bad carbs.

Why Some Carbs Are Different from Others

As you learned in Chapter 2, it isn't all carbs that are making Americans obese; it's the so-called refined ones, mainly flour products, potatoes, rice, and sugar. What exactly is it about these foods that makes people gain weight? Let's go back to basic nutrition for a minute.

There are three distinct kinds of food: fat, protein, and carbohydrates. Each has its own building block.

Fat is composed of fatty acids, protein of amino acids, and carbohydrates of glucose. Most of the fat in our diet comes from the fatty parts of meat, dairy products, and oily fruits and vegetables like nuts and olives. We get protein from eggs, dairy products, the lean parts of meat, nuts, beans, and protein-rich vegetables. Carbohydrates are plant products like fruits, vegetables, grains, potatoes, and sugar.

Before any of these foods can pass through the walls of your intestine into your bloodstream, your digestive tract has to sever the bonds that hold their molecules together and turn them back into their original building blocks. As food inches its way down your intestine, your digestive juices break down fat to fatty acids, protein to amino acids, and carbohydrate to glucose, the forms in which they enter your bloodstream.

"Glucose Shocks"

Considering that all carbohydrates eventually break down to glucose, what difference does it make whether they're in the form of fruit, vegetables, starch, or sugar when you eat them? Until recently, nutritionists made no distinction—"a carb is a carb," they used to say. However, it turns out there's a big difference in the way various carbohydrates affect your body, and that difference is the key to understanding why refined carbohydrates make people fat. It's also the key to losing weight without depriving yourself of satisfying amounts of good, healthful food.

The glucose molecules in carbohydrates are linked together end to end like railroad cars. It's the job of your digestive system to unhitch them so they can pass into your bloodstream. But

IN THEIR OWN WORDS

Name and Age: Linda, 50

Pounds Lost: 18 in 18 months

Health Benefits: Reduced cholesterol

"I fit into my daughter's little black cocktail dress!"

I had been at the same weight for so long, I had thrown away all my smaller-size dresses. A friend suggested I read *The Glycemic Load Diet*. The plan was easy to follow, so I stuck with it.

A couple of months later, when dressing for a party, I was surprised to find that all of my cocktail dresses were too big. In desperation, I grabbed a little black cocktail dress out of my petite, college-age daughter's closet. I fit into my daughter's little black cocktail dress! It just fit. Now all my clothes are too big!

I'll never give up this diet. This diet seems a lot easier to stay on, and I've made it a way of life.

Mother Nature doesn't give up her bounty easily. The glucose molecules of natural carbohydrates—whole fruits and vegetables—bond tightly to one another and intertwine with indigestible fiber and cellulose. Many fruits and vegetables contain natural "sugar-blocking" chemicals that deactivate digestive enzymes. Because of these inhibitors to digestion, it takes time for your digestive juices to unhitch the glucose molecules and free them up so they can be absorbed into your bloodstream. The glucose in these kinds of carbohydrates trickles into your system slowly, over the course of several hours.

It's a much different story for starchy carbohydrates like bread, potatoes, and rice. The bonds that hold their molecules together are much weaker and easily severed by digestive juices, and there's no indigestible fiber or cellulose to get in the way. As soon as these kinds of carbohydrates hit your digestive tract, their glucose molecules come unhitched and, within minutes, without having to travel more than a foot or two down your intestines, enter your bloodstream. Instead of slowly trickling into your system, as glucose in fresh fruit and vegetables does, the glucose in starch rushes into your bloodstream all at once. Within minutes, your blood glucose shoots up to levels never experienced by your prehistoric ancestors. These "glucose shocks" are foreign to the way human digestive systems worked for millions of years before starch came on the scene. It's not surprising that refined carbohydrates wreak havoc on the hormones that regulate body weight.

How Glucose Shocks Make You Gain Weight

Your pancreas secretes whatever amount of insulin it takes to keep your blood glucose levels in a safe range. That's easy to do when you eat the kind of food cave dwellers lived on—meat and fresh vegetation. Your pancreas only has to make enough insulin to handle small amounts of glucose that seep into your bloodstream over hours. But when you eat refined carbs, large amounts of glucose flood your bloodstream all at once and force your pancreas to secrete unnaturally large amounts of insulin. You make even more insulin if you have insulin resistance, in which case your pancreas has to secrete as much as six times more insulin than normal to get the job done. Over time, repeated glucose shocks can exhaust your pancreas and cause diabetes. They also encourage your body to store calories as fat.

Another problem with refined carbs is that they travel only a foot or two down your intestinal tract before they short-circuit into your bloodstream. Unlike other foods, they never get to the last part of your digestive tract, where certain appetite-suppressing hormones are produced. Normally, these hormones act as messengers to let your brain know your intestines have received enough food so you'll stop eating, but starch doesn't get far enough down your digestive tract to trigger them.

A particularly strange quality of starch is that you actually don't taste much of it. Only a small fraction of the starch you eat turns to glucose in your mouth, so you can taste it. Most of it passes into your stomach without interacting with your tastebuds. However, after it reaches your stomach, it immediately breaks down to sugar. This unusual quality of starch further encourages weight gain, because the less you taste the glucose you eat, the less it satisfies your appetite. When scientists fed glucose to subjects through tubes placed in their stomachs, it had much less of an appetite-satisfying effect than glucose taken by mouth.

All these attributes of starch promote overeating and obesity. In one research study, people who were fed starchy breakfasts and lunches consumed an astonishing 80 percent more calories in the afternoon and evening than subjects fed the same amount of calories in the form of omelets, fruits, and vegetables. The bottom line is that refined carbohydrates are unnatural foods that behave unnaturally in our bodies. It's not surprising that the more of these "bad carbs" we eat, the fatter and more diabetic we get.

The reason low-carb diets cause weight loss is not that they restrict carbohydrates in general. In fact, the more fruits and vegetables people consume, the less likely they are to be overweight. Low-carb diets work because they eliminate refined carbohydrates—flour products, potatoes, rice, and sugar.

Moving Beyond Atkins

Atkins was on the right track. His diet eliminated refined carbohydrates. The problem was, it restricted too many other foods. Most people just can't go very long without fruits, vegetables, and a few sweets. But Atkins was a man with a point to prove. After being called a charlatan in the 1970s, he was intent on proving that cutting carbs and continuing to eat fat and cholesterol could produce weight loss without raising blood cholesterol levels. He eventually proved his point, but his advice never changed much. His radical low-carb diet was essentially the same in the 1990s as it was when he first recommended it in the 1960s.

It's been more than 40 years since Atkins published his first book. Although junk science, diet hype, and academic turf battles have obscured the progress that has been made, medical science knows much more about metabolism and nutrition now than it did then.

- Twenty years ago, doctors didn't know about insulin resistance. Correcting this condition is the key to successful weight loss. Now that scientists have pinpointed the body chemistry disturbances that cause insulin resistance, it's possible to target diet, exercise, and medications, if necessary, toward relieving it.
- Nutritionists now know that only a few carbohydrates trigger excessive insulin secretion. Many of the foods the Atkins diet forbids—including fruits, vegetables, milk, and even sweets—prevent food cravings and can actually help you lose weight. The good news is that you only need to avoid a handful of bad carbs that aren't very tasty to begin with.
- Scientists have discovered that rapid weight loss triggers metabolic reactions that thwart further weight loss. Now you can take measures to counteract this diet-wrecking problem.
- Scientists have gained a much clearer understanding of what people need to do to keep their arteries healthy. With the right strategy, you can lose weight while at the same time lowering your risk of heart and artery disease.

Thanks to these and other new discoveries about nutrition and metabolism, it is now possible to harness the weight-loss power of low-carb dieting with a healthier, more enjoyable lifestyle that even people not endowed with unusual willpower can follow for life. The secret is in understanding something called the *glycemic load* and discovering how to activate your slow-twitch muscles, both of which you'll learn about in the next section of this book.

Part 2

The Glycemic Load Diet and Slow-Twitch Muscle Activation Plan

4

Lightening Your Glycemic Load: The Key to Easy Weight Loss

The reason most diets fail is simply that people can't stick with them. Low-fat diets are especially hard to follow. People crave the richness of fat and quickly either fall off the wagon or try to satisfy their hunger by eating too much starch and sugar. That's why low-fat diets require you to count calories—essentially to go hungry. Low-*carb* diets are easier to follow because you can eat satisfying amounts of food. However, they often make the mistake of restricting too many foods. Currently popular low-carb diets limit fruits, vegetables, dairy products, and sweets and usually can't resist throwing in some low-cholesterol advice. All these restrictions inevitably lead to food cravings and diet failure. However, most important, they divert attention from the real culprits: foods that raise your body's demands for insulin. As you learned in Chapter 3, the starch in refined carbohydrates causes your blood glucose to shoot up to levels never experienced by your prehistoric ancestors. These "glucose shocks" trigger excessive insulin secretion, which promotes fat accumulation.

Understanding Glycemic Indexes

It's difficult to predict whether a particular food will cause a glucose shock simply by measuring its carbohydrate content. Some carbs break down to glucose faster and raise insulin levels more than others do. Food scientists have learned that the best way to tell how high blood glucose goes after eating a food is to give a standardized amount to human subjects and measure their blood glucose levels afterward. Nutritionists now rate foods according to their *glycemic indexes,* the amount a food raises blood glucose compared with a benchmark—usually white bread. An apple, for example, has a glycemic index of 52, which means that 50 grams of carbohydrate in an apple raises blood glucose levels 52 percent as much as 50 grams of carbohydrate in white bread.

Why Glycemic Indexes Are Misleading

The discovery that some carbs raise blood glucose levels more than others do was good news for low-carb dieters. They didn't have to avoid all carbohydrates, only ones with high glycemic indexes. Soon, popular diet books such as *The South Beach Diet* and *The Glycemic Index Diet* published lists of glycemic indexes to help low-carb dieters avoid glucose shocks. However, while these lists increased awareness of differences among carbs, they also created misconceptions that have kept the low-carb eating style from realizing its potential. To see how misleading these measurements can be, look at the glycemic indexes of the following foods.

Glycemic Index (percentage compared with 50 grams of white bread)

Food	Glycemic Index
Tomatoes	23
Spaghetti	64
Carrots	68
White bread	100
Bagel	103

If you keep in mind that foods rated less than 55 are considered "low" on the glycemic index scale, you will conclude, correctly, that you don't have to worry as much about tomatoes as you do about bagels, even though both are carbohydrates. However, notice that carrots, which you probably thought were good for you, have a higher glycemic index than spaghetti, a notoriously starchy food. That doesn't sound right, does it?

The Devil in the Details: Serving Size

It's important to understand that glycemic indexes are raw laboratory measurements. The researchers who reported these numbers warned against using them *without correcting for the amounts people typically eat*. That may seem like a mundane technicality, but it makes a world of difference in the way you need to eat to avoid glucose shocks. Here's why glycemic indexes, which are not adjusted for serving size, are so misleading.

To measure the glycemic index of a food, scientists have to feed volunteers enough of it to provide a standard amount of carbohydrate available for absorption into the bloodstream; researchers have chosen 50 grams as the standard. However, the amount of available carbohydrate in various plant-based foods varies tremendously. For example, because carrots contain so much water and unavailable carbohydrate in the form of indigestible fiber, to provide 50 grams of available carbohydrate, researchers had to feed each subject *seven* full-size carrots. In contrast, to provide 50 grams of available carbohydrate in spaghetti, they had to feed subjects only a cupful. Of course, most people don't eat seven carrots in one sitting, but they often eat a cupful of spaghetti or more. The reason glycemic indexes are misleading is that the amounts researchers have to feed subjects to get 50 grams of available carbohydrate bear little resemblance to the amounts people typically eat. The glycemic indexes of many fruits and vegetables, like carrots, turn out to be as high as those of many starchy carbohydrates, like spaghetti.

Missing Out on the Good Carbs and Not Recognizing the Bad

The failure of popular diet books to correct glycemic indexes for serving size caused a lot of people to deprive themselves of healthful foods, including many fruits and vegetables, they didn't need to avoid. Research studies consistently show that the more

IN THEIR OWN WORDS

Name and Age: Bert, 60

Pounds Lost: 30 in 12 months

Health Benefits: Lost 5 inches off waist, achieved steadier energy levels, improved digestive health

"I weigh the same now as when I played high school football!"

I'm one of those ex–football jocks who put on weight. I've always exercised, and I'm in pretty good aerobic shape. I just couldn't lose my paunch. I've gone on a lot of low-calorie diets, but I got tired of walking around hungry all the time.

What's different about the Glycemic Load Diet is that it is not a typical fad diet. It's a style of eating that you can stay on forever. I'm never hungry, but I lost 30 pounds in a year. I frequently eat out for business. The diet is quite easy to follow in restaurants: You order a nice big dinner with a little dessert. You eat everything, but you make a little starch pile just like Dr. Thompson suggests.

I weigh the same now as when I played high school football! I don't have cravings. I don't feel deprived. I eat better than ever.

fruits and vegetables people eat, the less obesity, diabetes, and heart disease they have. Natural inhibitors of glucose absorption in fruits and vegetables prevent glucose shocks and reduce hunger without adding calories. Also, meals require adequate volume to be satisfying, and fruits and vegetables provide more volume than other foods but with fewer calories. Take it from a doctor who's been treating overweight patients for 25 years: People don't get fat eating carrots.

But here's what's even more deceptive about glycemic indexes: They give the impression that starchy foods like bread and spaghetti are only a little worse than fruits and vegetables. In fact, as you will see, they are much worse.

Getting It Right: Glycemic Loads

Food scientists have recently developed a way to correct glycemic indexes for serving size. It's called the *glycemic load,* and it represents the effects on blood glucose of amounts of food people actually eat, rather than what goes on in the research lab. I can't overemphasize the importance of using glycemic loads instead of glycemic indexes. It changes the whole approach to avoiding glucose shocks. To understand why, consider the glycemic loads of the same five foods we looked at previously. Notice that this list specifies typical serving sizes: The glycemic load represents the percentage a typical helping of each food raises blood sugar compared with that of one slice of white bread.

Food (serving size)	*Glycemic Load (percentage compared with a 1-ounce slice of white bread)*
Carrot (1 medium, 8" length)	11
Tomato (1 medium)	15
White bread (1 slice, ⅜" thick)	100
Spaghetti (1 c)	166
Bagel (1 medium)	340

Makes more sense, doesn't it? The rabbit food is at one end of the scale, the starchy stuff at the other. You can see why glycemic loads allow you to enjoy foods you might avoid if you let glycemic indexes be your guide.

But here's what's more important: Correcting glycemic indexes for serving size exposes refined carbs as the culprits they really are. Bagels, for example, aren't just a little worse than carrots, they're terrible! You would have to eat 30 raw carrots to get the glucose shock you get from one bagel. Table 4.1 provides a list of

Table 4.1 Glycemic Loads of Common Foods

(*Note:* Many of the glycemic load lists published in books, in the medical literature, and on the Internet randomly assign a slice of white bread a glycemic load of 10 instead of 100. You can convert those values to the ones here by multiplying by 10. The glycemic loads listed here have also been corrected for typical American serving sizes, which sometimes differ from ones derived in other countries.)

Food Item	Description	Typical Serving	Glycemic Load
Pancake	5" diameter	2½ oz	346
Bagel	1 medium	3⅓ oz	340
Orange soda	8 oz glass	12 oz	314
White rice	1 c	6½ oz	283
White bread	2 slices, ⅜" thick	2¾ oz	260
Baked potato	1 medium	5 oz	246
Whole wheat bread	2 slices, ⅜" thick	2¾ oz	234
Raisin bran	1 c	2 oz	227
Brown rice	1 c	6½ oz	222
French fries	Medium serving, McDonald's	5¼ oz	219
Coca-Cola	12 oz can	12 oz	218
Hamburger bun	5" diameter	2½ oz	213
English muffin	1 medium	2 oz	208
Doughnut	1 medium	2 oz	205
Cornflakes	1 c	1 oz	199
Macaroni	1 c	5 oz	181
Corn on the cob	1 ear	5⅓ oz	171
Blueberry muffin	2½" diameter	2 oz	169
Spaghetti	1 c	5 oz	166
Instant oatmeal (cooked)	1 c	8 oz	154
Chocolate cake	1 slice (4" × 4" × 1")	3 oz	154
Grape-Nuts	1 c	1 oz	142
Cheerios	1 c	1 oz	142
Special K	1 c	1 oz	133
Tortilla, corn	1 medium	1¾ oz	120
Orange juice	8 oz glass	8 oz	119
Cookie (lab standard, 30 g)	1 medium	1 oz	114
Grapefruit juice, unsweetened	8 oz glass	8 oz	100
White bread	1 thin slice, ¼" thick	1 1/16 oz	100
Banana	1 medium	3¼ oz	85
All-Bran	½ c	1 oz	85
Tortilla, wheat	1 medium	1¾ oz	80
Apple	1 medium	5½ oz	78

Food Item	Description	Typical Serving	Glycemic Load
Orange	1 medium	6 oz	71
Pinto beans	½ c	3 oz	57
Pear	1 medium	6 oz	57
Pineapple	1 slice (¾" × 3½")	3 oz	50
Peach	1 medium	4 oz	47
Grapes	1 c (40 grapes)	2½ oz	47
Kidney beans	½ c	3 oz	40
Grapefruit	1 half	4½ oz	32
Table sugar	1 rounded tsp	⅙ oz	28
Milk (whole)	8 oz glass	8 oz	27
Peas	¼ c	1½ oz	16
Tomato	1 medium	5 oz	15
Strawberries	1 c	5½ oz	13
Carrot (raw)	1 medium (7½" length)	3 oz	11
Peanuts	¼ c	1¼ oz	7
Spinach	1 c	2½ oz	<15
Pork	Two 5 oz chops	10 oz	<15
Margarine	1 pat	¼ oz	<15
Lettuce	1 c	2½ oz	<15
Fish	8 oz fillet	8 oz	<15
Eggs	1 egg	1½ oz	<15
Cucumber	1 c	6 oz	<15
Chicken	1 breast	10 oz	<15
Cheese	1 slice (2" × 2" × 1")	2 oz	<15
Butter	1 Tbsp	¼ oz	<15
Broccoli	½ c	1½ oz	<15
Beef	10 oz steak	10 oz	<15

the glycemic loads of typical servings of some common foods. (You'll find a more complete list in Appendix A, page 330.)

How low should your daily glycemic load be? To stop your body from overproducing insulin, you need to keep your daily tally less than about 500. Generally, individual foods with ratings under 100 are okay; most people can eat satisfying amounts of these without gaining weight or raising their risk of diabetes. However, more than a couple of servings a day of foods with higher ratings are likely to drive up insulin levels, encourage weight gain, and raise the risk of diabetes.

Reducing Your Glycemic Load: A Simple Plan for Effective Weight Loss

All this glycemic load business sounds very scientific, but if you look twice at the list of glycemic loads in Table 4.1 on page 48, you can see what's going on. The culprits stand out in sharp relief. The foods with the highest glycemic loads (greater than 100) are ones most people would call "starchy"—grain products, potatoes, and rice—and soft drinks. Indeed, those are the main sources of glucose shocks in the American diet. According to the Nurses' Health Study, an analysis of the dietary habits of 17,000 American nurses, the combined cumulative glycemic loads of grain products, potatoes, and rice in the typical American's diet are equal to more than *20 times* the total glycemic load of any other food, including sugar and candy. That's the *average* consumption. The same study showed that women who developed diabetes ate significantly *more* than average amounts of those foods.

Now you know what you need to do. If you get rid of just four foods—flour products, potatoes, rice, and soft drinks—the glycemic load of your diet will be a fraction of what it was. You don't even need a list of glycemic loads to tell you what to eat. Starch is never hidden or blended into other foods. You can see it from across the room. The culprits are even color-coded for you: They're usually *white*. The only other foods with glycemic loads as high as the starchy stuff are juices and soft drinks. So, if you cut out the starch and sugar-containing beverages, you eliminate nearly all of the glucose shocks in your diet. Taking into account the minor glycemic loads you get from other carbohydrates you might eat, you can usually get away with eating the equivalent of about one full serving of starch a day.

Here's my advice: Forget about lists. Just don't eat more than a third of a serving of flour products, potatoes, or rice at any meal, and abstain from sugar-containing soft drinks and fruit juices. Otherwise, eat anything you want. There's probably not enough starch or sugar in the rest of your food to cause you trouble. A weight-loss program can't get any simpler than that, which is why this will finally be the weight loss program that works for you.

Opening the Door to a Richer, More Flavorful Way of Eating

The strict low-carb diets of the Atkins era went further than they needed to in restricting fruits, vegetables, and sweets and even dairy products but not far enough in eliminating starch. Certainly, you can shed pounds faster if you eliminate all carbs, but that weight loss comes at a high price in terms of satisfaction and healthiness. Such diets create irresistible food cravings. Most people just can't stay with them for long. To make up for restricting so many nutritious foods, many diets recommend taking vitamins, stool softeners, and various supplements. This is unnecessary if you eliminate only refined carbohydrates. No one in the history of the world has ever suffered any medical condition caused by lack of starch.

There's another bonus to reducing the glycemic load of your diet. Because starch is essentially tasteless, when you eliminate it, you remove little in the way of taste and texture, and you make room for more delicious food. Starch no longer dilutes the flavors in your diet. Instead of filling up on the same bland staples at every meal, you branch out to more flavor and richness. Eliminating starch allows you to enjoy the pleasing qualities of a wider variety of foods. Don't be surprised if you find yourself eating better than you were before!

5

Job One: Purge Starch from Your Diet

Now you know why starch is public enemy number one. As soon as it hits your digestive tract, it turns to sugar and floods your bloodstream with glucose. These glucose shocks cause your pancreas to secrete excessive amounts of insulin, a notoriously obesity-promoting hormone. In this chapter, I'm going to pass on some tricks that will make eliminating glucose shocks and reducing your daily glycemic load easy for you.

Some of the advice I'm going to give you is based on my experience not only as a doctor but also as a patient. As a cardiologist, I followed the party line for years. I avoided cholesterol and ate plenty of refined carbohydrates. In 1999, I found out I had type 1 diabetes. As a doctor, I was well acquainted with the complications of poorly controlled diabetes, such as eye, kidney, and blood vessel damage. Discovering I had this problem was akin to someone holding a gun to my head and telling me to keep my blood sugar down.

How I Became a Human Glycemic Load Meter

The first thing I did when I discovered I had diabetes was buy a monitoring device so I could measure my blood glucose levels at home. In the past 12 years, I have checked my blood sugar thousands of times, after every kind of meal, snack, and physical activity. I can personally attest to the importance of the glycemic load ratings. My blood glucose levels directly reflect the glycemic loads of the foods I eat. As long as I avoid foods with high glycemic loads, my blood levels are fine. I don't have to think of much else. I can eat a full-course dinner of meat, vegetables, and salad, and my blood sugar hardly rises at all. I can even have some candy for dessert, and it still doesn't go up too much. However, if I eat so much as a single slice of bread or some potatoes, it skyrockets.

My low-glycemic-load eating style has been effective for preventing glucose surges and for losing weight. From my blood tests, no one could tell I am diabetic, and I got rid of 20 pounds I needed to lose. The amazing thing is, I don't feel like I'm dieting or depriving myself at all. I avoid bread, potatoes, rice, and soft drinks, but for the most part eat what I want.

Although I've never displayed much discipline when it comes to eating, I have not found lowering my glycemic load difficult to do. Truthfully, I eat better now than I did before. I assure you, a low-glycemic-load diet is a way of eating you can continue for life, even if you are not endowed with unusual willpower. I do it, my patients do it, and you can do it, too.

Strategies for Eliminating "Starchy Fillers"

The secret to eliminating glucose shocks is to "pick the low-lying fruit": Concentrate on what reaps the most benefit with the least effort. Without question, the biggest bang for your buck—in fact, almost all the bang—comes from reducing your intake of what I call starchy fillers: bread, potatoes, and rice side dishes. These are by far the major offenders in most people's diets.

As deeply ingrained as the starch-with-every-meal habit is, starchy fillers are where we get most of our glucose shocks. The good news is that these are the easiest foods to eliminate. They're usually served as side dishes, not intended to be the highlight of meals. You don't miss out on any delicious entrées or draw attention to yourself by passing up the bread plate or leaving some potatoes on your plate. Because starch is mainly tasteless, when you remove it, you remove little in the way of flavor from your diet.

You also remove nothing in the way of essential vitamins, minerals, or fiber. This fact is important to remember, because diets deficient in vital nutrients inevitably trigger cravings for what's missing. However, bread, potatoes, and rice contain nothing you can't live without. There is no such thing as a starch deficiency. Humans existed for millions of years without it, and our prehistoric ancestors were taller, stronger, and less susceptible to many diseases before starchy carbohydrates came on the scene.

Keep in mind that this is not a calorie-restricted diet. You shouldn't even call it a diet. It's a way to avoid a substance that is toxic to you if you have insulin resistance, which you probably do if you are overweight. You can eat virtually everything else— meat, dairy products, nuts, fresh fruit, vegetables, even a little candy—and you can eat until you're satisfied. In fact, you don't even have to swear off bread, potatoes, and rice entirely. Just limit yourself to no more than a third of a typical serving at any meal, or the equivalent of approximately one average-size helping a day.

Step 1: Pass Up the Bread Plate

No food is more deeply ingrained in American and European dietary tradition than bread. "Breaking bread" is synonymous with dining itself. It's part of religious rituals. We expect it with virtually every meal. But the plain truth is, our devotion to bread is killing us. You might recall from Chapter 2 that the skyrocketing obesity and diabetes rates in America in the last

40 years correlate precisely with our rising consumption of wheat products. The average American gets 5 to 10 times more glucose shocks from bread and baked goods than from any other single food.

So don't fall for the old trick restaurants play of enticing you to fill up on bread before the main dish arrives. Your first bite of food at a meal should never be a refined carbohydrate. When your stomach is empty, starch goes directly into your bloodstream and causes a huge glucose shock. If you want something to eat before the main dish arrives, have some real food—soup, salad, or an appetizer.

If occasionally you can't resist having some bread, wait until you finish the rest of your meal. That will allow time for the other foods to reach the appetite centers in your brain, and the fat and fiber in your meal will slow the entry of glucose into your bloodstream. Then eat just a little, a half slice at the most. Roll it around in your mouth a while before you swallow it. The longer your saliva works on it, the more glucose it releases in your mouth instead of your stomach, the more it stimulates your tastebuds, and the more it will satisfy whatever craving you have for it. Put some butter or margarine on it if you want; this isn't a low-fat diet.

The reality is, if you are serious about eliminating glucose shocks, you must eliminate bread in all forms: rolls, bagels, muffins, scones, crackers, sandwich bread, hamburger buns, and crusts. This is central to reducing the glycemic load of your diet. The good news is, if your diet is typical of what most Americans eat, that's almost *all* you have to do. The rest is easy.

The Whole Grain Myth: What about whole wheat bread? Isn't that supposed to be good for you? Indeed, real whole grain bread—bread that contains whole kernels of grain—has more vitamins, protein, and fiber than white bread does. Unfortunately, though, when it comes to causing glucose shocks, a slice of whole grain bread is just as bad as—in fact, slightly worse than—a slice of white bread.

Indeed, whole grain bread breaks down to glucose slower than white bread does, so its glycemic index (not load) is a little lower. However, those tiny kernels are packed with starch. Slice for slice, whole grain bread contains up to twice as much starch as white bread. You simply get more food in a slice of whole grain bread. The glycemic load of whole grain bread—which takes into account the amount of carbohydrate in a typical serving—is actually higher than that of white bread.

Actually, if you ate the same amount of carbohydrate in the form of whole grain bread as you did in white bread, you would, in fact, modestly reduce the glycemic load. But because whole grain bread simply contains more food per slice than white bread, that would mean eating fewer or smaller slices. If you just substitute whole grain for white bread without reducing the size or the number of the slices, you end up getting a larger glucose shock and more calories to boot.

As it turns out, the modest reductions in glycemic index (not load) that researchers have reported for whole grain breads are, in fact, for breads much higher in kernel content than the ones you're likely to find in a grocery store. Kernels accounted for 80 percent of the weight of the breads the researchers called "whole grain" but make up less than 20 percent of most commercially available whole grain breads. Brown bread, rye bread, and so-called whole wheat (as opposed to whole grain) bread contain less than 5 percent kernels.

Why don't supermarkets sell breads with higher kernel contents? It's a matter of palatability. Our ancestors learned thousands of years ago that the husks of grains have to be removed and the starchy cores pulverized to make them edible. A television journalist recently asked an owner of a bread company why manufacturers don't market breads with higher kernel contents. The company owner replied that people don't want bread that "tastes like cardboard."

What about studies showing that people who eat whole grain bread are healthier than folks who eat white bread? Whole grain consumption is a sign of someone who tries to live healthily. It doesn't mean whole grain bread does them any good.

The Fiber Factor: One reason whole grain bread has a reputation for being healthful is that the husks of wheat kernels contain insoluble fiber, an indigestible carbohydrate that helps prevent constipation and other colon problems. Indeed, the diets of most Americans and Europeans are grossly deficient in this kind of fiber. However, there isn't enough insoluble fiber in most whole grain breads to make much of a difference—certainly not enough to make up for the glucose shocks you get. The recommended daily requirement for insoluble fiber is about 20 grams; a slice of whole grain bread contains about 2 grams. By comparison, half a cup of bran cereal provides 14 grams. You're better off getting your fiber from fruits, vegetables, and bran cereal than from bread.

Step 2: Push Aside the Potatoes and Rice

Imagine a pile of sugar on your plate the size of a baked potato or a serving of rice. The effect on your blood insulin levels is the same. If you want to eliminate glucose shocks, you have to reduce your consumption of potatoes and rice.

Perhaps you're thinking that rice must be okay because Asians eat a lot of it and they're not as fat as Americans and Europeans are. Indeed, Asians have been eating rice for thousands of years. However, until the 20th century, they consumed only small amounts of it. Rice kernels are difficult to extract from their husks. People had to grind it between stones and pick out the kernels by hand. Only the rich could afford to eat much of it. Only after the advent of rice-polishing machines in the 1920s did most Asians begin eating large amounts of the stuff. Now they, too, are overweight. Asia has the fastest-rising incidence of obesity and diabetes in the world.

The trick to reducing your potato and rice consumption is to have a few bites if you must, but don't use them to satisfy your appetite. Wait until you finish eating the other food on your plate, then go ahead and take a few bites. You will find you need only a little—probably less than a fourth of a typical serving. Keep in mind as you eat these starches that even though they're largely tasteless, you might as well be eating sugar.

Step 3: Learn Ways to Reduce the Glucose Shocks in Starchy Main Dishes

Avoiding starchy side dishes like bread, potatoes, and rice is easy enough. They're extras; you're not obliged to eat them. But what about the starch in main dishes like hamburgers, pizza, and pasta? Does eliminating starch mean you can't share meals with friends or eat in your favorite restaurants? Do you have to consult a food guide to find out how much starch is in the dishes you eat?

Interestingly enough, starch is rarely concealed. It's always right out in plain sight. There's no problem spotting the starch in a hamburger or piece of pizza. It's in the bun and crust. Moreover, starch is rarely blended with other ingredients. You can usually separate it from the rest of the dish with a few strokes of a knife and fork.

The plain visibility and separateness of starch from other components of dishes reflects its distinct physical properties and the way it behaves in food preparation. In contrast, fat is usually invisible and blended with other ingredients. You have to consult a fat-gram counter to tell how much fat is in a dish, and once it's added, it usually can't be removed. One of the reasons low-carb diets are more effective than low-fat diets is that the culprits are so obvious. It's much simpler to avoid starch than fat. Here are some tricks for reducing the glycemic loads of starch-containing main courses.

Build a Starch Pile: Because the starchy parts of dishes are often easy to see and separate from other ingredients, you can usually pick them out as you eat. A good technique for reducing the glycemic load of your meals is to build a pile on the side of your plate with the starch you remove from your food. Granted, starch is part of the appeal of some dishes. However, you can usually enjoy those dishes while eating a fraction of the starch they're served with if you simply pick some of the starch out as you eat and put it on your starch pile. After you finish the rest of your meal, if you still want some starch, you can take it from the pile. However, by then the other food will have had time to reach the appetite centers in your brain, and you won't be so ravenous.

You'll probably find that seeing all that starch in a pile dampens your enthusiasm for it. As you leave the table, you can congratulate yourself on the size of the pile you left behind.

Use Other Foods to Slow the Absorption of Starch: When you can't avoid starch, you can cushion the glucose shock it causes by paying attention to the foods you eat with it and the order in which you eat them. Having other food in your stomach before eating refined carbohydrates reduces the size of the resulting glucose surge. Fat slows the digestion of starch, and fiber in fruits and vegetables acts like a kind of sponge, soaking up glucose and slowing its entry into your bloodstream. That's why it's smart to eat a salad before a meal and to avoid eating starch or sugar on an empty stomach.

One of the best ways to reduce your glycemic load is to eat nuts. You can enjoy these immensely satisfying morsels any time you want. Nuts—any kind of nuts—are full of vitamins, minerals, fiber, protein, and omega-3 fatty acids, and they contain virtually no starch. Their glycemic loads are negligible. A couple of handfuls of nuts before a meal will slow stomach emptying so you stay full longer and help keep other foods from raising your blood sugar.

Nuts are probably the most natural food you can eat. Humans have been eating them for millions of years. Adding nuts to your diet might actually help you lose weight.

Learn to Make Wraps instead of Sandwiches: Putting meat or cheese between slices of bread is a good way to make expensive food go further, but sandwiches are a major source of glucose shocks. Although they're a popular lunch food, there are plenty of alternatives. A salad with lots of rich ingredients—such as meat, cheese, and nuts—will fill you up without causing a glucose shock. Most soups are fine if you leave some of the potatoes and noodles in the bowl. Soups and salads aren't as easy to pack for work as sandwiches are, but you can do it with plastic containers and a thermos bottle.

One reason sandwiches are so popular is that you can pick them up with your hands and eat them; you don't need a plate, knife, or fork. If you want the convenience of a sandwich without all that bread, learn to make a wrap, a sandwich made with a tortilla instead of bread. Just wrap up your ingredients in a tortilla, fold the bottom so they don't fall out, and eat away. A wheat tortilla has a glycemic load of 80, compared with 260 for two slices of white bread. If you use low-carb tortillas, the glycemic load is negligible.

Eat More Burger and Less Bun: Another major source of glucose shocks is hamburger buns (glycemic load of 213). Try skipping the bun altogether. You'll be surprised at how much better a piece of hamburger topped with all the extras is without the bread dough to dilute its taste. These days, restaurants are accustomed to serving burgers this way.

If you have to have some bun with your burger, you can reduce the glucose shock to an acceptable level by removing the top bun. There are two ways you can do that: Either take off the top bun and eat your burger with a knife and fork, or hold the burger in your hands and peel away the top bun, chunk by chunk, as you eat.

You can also make a good hamburger with a tortilla. Cut the hamburger patty in half and wrap it in a tortilla with all the extras. Tortillas also make good substitutes for hot dog buns. The high fiber content of low-carb tortillas soaks up fat from the meat, which moistens the tortilla and brings out a pleasing flavor.

Eat Your Pasta al Dente with Plenty of Amendments: Make no mistake, pasta is full of starch, and if you're trying to get rid of glucose shocks, you need to eat it sparingly. Fortunately, most of us don't eat pasta with every meal, as we do bread, potatoes, and rice. Pasta also has some redeeming qualities that lessen its impact on your blood glucose. The starch in pasta turns to glucose in your intestinal tract a little more slowly than does the starch in other flour products, such as bread. Pasta's effects on your blood glucose level also depend on how you prepare it. The more you cook it, the faster it will break down to glucose in your digestive tract, and the more it will raise your blood glucose level. You can reduce the size of the glucose shock by eating pasta *al dente*—cooked less so it has a firmer texture. The glycemic load of a cup of spaghetti boiled 10 to 15 minutes is 166. If you boil it for 20 minutes, the glycemic load goes up to 213.

Another redeeming quality of pasta is that you can mix it with other ingredients, such as vegetables, meat, and olive oil, and the more of the other ingredients you eat, the less pasta you need to satisfy your hunger. In addition, the fat in meat and the fiber in vegetables slow the digestion of starch.

Whole grain pastas generally have lower glycemic loads than regular pastas. For example, a cup of whole grain spaghetti has a glycemic load of 126, compared with 166 for an equal-size serving of regular spaghetti. However, for most pasta lovers, the modest benefit of switching to whole grain doesn't make up for the sacrifice of taste and texture.

Learn to Remove Starch from Dishes After They're Served: If you remove the outer 2 inches of crust from a slice of pizza, you avoid about three-fourths of the bread. Just stick your knife under the topping, cut away a couple of inches of crust, and put it on your starch pile. That will leave enough crust to provide a small piece to go along with each bite of topping. The glycemic load of the remaining quarter-slice of crust is only about 20, not enough to cause a glucose shock, even if you have two or three slices.

Most casseroles are easy to handle. You can pluck out the potatoes or crust and put them on your starch pile. Rice casseroles are tougher. The best way to handle them is to serve yourself less rice and more of the amendments and push some of the rice to the side of your plate as you eat. Sometimes you have to be content with just lowering the amount of starch you get in entrées and not eliminating it. If your diet is typical, getting rid of the starchy fillers—the bread, potato, and rice side dishes—will get rid of most of the glucose shocks. If you just reduce the starch in main dishes by, say, half, and avoid the starchy side dishes, the glycemic load of your diet will be a fraction of what it was.

Forget What You Saw on Television about Breakfast Cereals:
Imagine you could make a food from the cheapest ingredients on Earth and obtain a patent that gave you exclusive rights to sell it. Without competition, you could make a large profit—that is, if you could convince people to buy it. The best way to do that? Advertise.

The fact is, you have been brainwashed. From the time you were old enough to sit in front of a television set, you were inundated by ads touting the deliciousness, health benefits, and fun to be had from eating breakfast cereals. Manufacturers put toys in cereal boxes to entice you. It only took a decade for television to change what we Americans ate for breakfast. We went from eating bacon and eggs to Wheaties and Cheerios. A generation of Americans grew up thinking cereals are "The Breakfast of Champions."

As convenient as breakfast cereals are, if you're trying to avoid glucose shocks, they're a terrible way to start the day. They're made from grain, the most concentrated source of starch known, and a lot of them are laced with sugar to boot. Most cereals have unacceptable glycemic loads, including ones touted on television for their health benefits, such as granola, Cheerios, raisin bran, and oatmeal. To make matters worse, we usually eat them in the morning, which is when our bodies are least able to handle carbohydrates without overproducing insulin. Starting the day with a glucose shock practically guarantees that you're going to eat more during the rest of the day. In one study, people who were fed instant oatmeal for breakfast consumed 80 percent more calories later in the day than did subjects fed omelets. Table 5.1 includes the glycemic loads of several popular breakfast cereals. Remember, anything over 100 will give you glucose shock.

The Benefits of Wheat Bran: Fiber is the part of fruits and vegetables that your digestive system doesn't break down and absorb. It travels through your digestive tract and out intact in your stool. There are two kinds, soluble and insoluble. Each has its own health benefits. Soluble fiber acts like a sponge and soaks up sugar and fat, delaying their entry into your bloodstream. This kind of fiber reduces the glycemic load of other

Table 5.1 Glycemic Loads of Popular Breakfast Cereals

Cereal	Serving Size	Glycemic Load
All-Bran	½ c	85
Muesli	1 c	95
Special K	1 c	133
Cheerios	1 c	142
Shredded wheat	1 c	142
Grape-Nuts	1 c	142
Puffed wheat	1 c	151
Instant oatmeal	1 c	154
Cream of Wheat	1 c	154
Total	1 c	161
Cornflakes	1 c	199
Rice Krispies	1 c	208
Rice Chex	1 c	218
Raisin bran	1 c	227

foods eaten with it, and is believed to help prevent obesity, diabetes, and gallbladder disease. Fruits and vegetables contain lots of soluble fiber.

Insoluble fiber works differently. It passes through your digestive tract as solid particles. This kind of fiber is valuable because it helps maintain normal bowel function. It's especially useful in relieving irritable bowel syndrome, a condition most of us suffer from at times, characterized by alternating constipation and diarrhea, pelletlike stools, and uncomfortable gas. Insoluble fiber also helps prevent more serious bowel problems, including diverticulitis and hemorrhoids. Because insoluble fiber provides bulk for the digestive tract to work on, many experts think that lack of it promotes overeating.

In the Western diet, insoluble fiber is harder to come by than the soluble kind. Prehistoric humans consumed huge amounts of it in grasses, roots, and unripe vegetation, but little remains in the modern diet. Consequently, diseases related to insoluble fiber deficiency have become increasingly common.

Although fruits and vegetables contain some insoluble fiber—mainly in their skins—we often don't eat enough for good bowel health. By far the most concentrated source of insoluble fiber in the Western diet happens to be the husk of the dreaded wheat kernel, the "bran." But don't rush to the grocery store to buy whole grain bread. Modern milling techniques remove almost all of the bran from wheat products, so most of the flour-based foods we eat are practically devoid of insoluble fiber. Even whole grain bread falls woefully short of providing adequate amounts.

One of the best ways to make sure you're getting enough insoluble fiber is to eat a high-fiber breakfast cereal. The problem is that few breakfast cereals come close to providing enough insoluble fiber to justify the glucose shocks they cause. The only exceptions are 100 percent bran cereals, such as All-Bran. The glycemic load of a half cup of All-Bran cereal is 85, not quite enough to cause a glucose shock but enough to help make sure you're getting adequate insoluble fiber.

Table 5.2 lists the insoluble fiber contents of several popular breakfast cereals. Notice that many cereals touted as being high in fiber don't come close to providing as much fiber as All-Bran cereal does.

Be careful not to equate oat bran with wheat bran. Oat bran is a good source of soluble fiber but provides little *in*soluble fiber. It can actually worsen the symptoms of irritable colon (or bowel) syndrome.

Table 5.2 Insoluble Fiber Content of Breakfast Cereals

Cereal	Serving Size	Insoluble Fiber (grams)
All-Bran	½ c	14
Fiber One	½ c	13
Bran Buds	⅓ c	10
Bran flakes	1 c	6
Oat bran	⅓ c	4
Raisin bran	½ c	3
Cheerios	1 c	2
Grape-Nuts	1 c	2
Oatmeal	1 c	2
Total	1 c	2
Wheaties	1 c	2
Rice Krispies	1 c	1
Cornflakes	1 c	1

IN THEIR OWN WORDS

Name and Age: Lisa, 47

Pounds Lost: 17 in 2 months

Health Benefits: Gained energy and mental sharpness; is no longer shaky when hungry

"It was truly effortless!"

I've tried the South Beach Diet, Weight Watchers, and a bunch of other diets, but I could never stay on them for long. Following the advice in the book is the easiest weight-loss program I have ever been on. I lost 17 pounds in 2 months, and it was truly effortless. My clothes fit better!

I used to obsess about food. But on this program, I didn't think I was being deprived of good-tasting food. I don't have food cravings anymore. I definitely noticed more energy. I am mentally sharper. The shakiness I got when I hadn't eaten for a while went away. My nervous system feels more stable.

Admittedly, 100 percent bran cereal is not most people's idea of exciting food. Some people think it tastes like cardboard. What's missing is fat and protein. You can turn bran cereal into a heartier breakfast by adding a handful of chopped walnuts and livening up its taste with some fruit or a couple of tablespoons of another breakfast cereal. Keep in mind that you don't have to have it for breakfast—you can eat it as a snack anytime.

What about bran muffins? Unfortunately, most commercially available bran muffins contain enough refined flour and sugar to cause a sizable glucose shock, and they don't provide nearly as much insoluble fiber as a serving of bran cereal. However, you can make your own high-fiber muffins by using less flour and more bran. You will find a recipe for low-glycemic-load, high-fiber muffins on page 173. One of those muffins will provide almost as much fiber as a bowl of bran cereal.

Don't Start Your Day with a Glucose Shock: Our bodies are particularly prone to glucose shocks in the morning. When you eat starchy cereals or baked goods for breakfast, your blood glucose skyrockets and then crashes about 4 hours later, often causing symptoms of hypoglycemia such as tiredness, poor concentration, and exaggerated hunger. Starting the day with a glucose shock also makes you want to eat more later in the day. Researchers demonstrated this by feeding experimental subjects starchy breakfasts and comparing their food intake with that of a group fed an equal number of calories in low-starch breakfasts. Over the course of a week, those who ate the starchier breakfasts consumed 145 more calories at lunch and dinner than those who ate the less starchy ones. That's enough to make you gain 60 pounds in 5 years. It really is true: You're better off eating bacon and eggs.

6

Eliminate Sugar-Sweetened Beverages

uestion: What's the easiest way to lose weight?
Answer: Eliminate sugar-containing beverages.

Let me explain. Sugar in liquids behaves much differently in your body than sugar in solids does. In solid form, such as in candy, sugar interacts with your tastebuds as you chew it, and it melts in your mouth. Tasting it has an appetite-suppressing effect. However, in liquids, most of the sugar flows past your tastebuds without stimulating them, which has much less of an appetite-satisfying effect. In one study, researchers fed sugar in the form of jelly beans to a group of subjects and sugar in a beverage to another group and then observed their food consumption afterward. The subjects who ate sugar in the jelly beans curtailed their intake of other foods by approximately as many calories as were in the jelly beans, as you would expect. However, the subjects who consumed sugar in beverage form didn't reduce their subsequent calorie consumption at all. In other words, sugar in liquids adds to calories from other foods rather than replaces them. Honestly, does drinking a Coke make you eat fewer french fries?

This is actually great news for dieters. If sugar-containing beverages provide no appetite-satisfying effects, *then getting rid of them won't increase your appetite.* That means you can eliminate a major source of calories without increasing your hunger for other foods. People are often amazed at the ease with which they lose weight when they just stop drinking sugar-containing beverages. Not only does sugar in liquids behave differently from sugar in solids in your mouth, it also acts differently in your stomach. After candy gets to your stomach, it has to wait its turn before it can pass into your intestine and be absorbed into your bloodstream. In the meantime, it mixes with other foods, which slows its digestion. However, sugar dissolved in liquids flows right around the other foods in your stomach, passes into your intestine, and releases glucose directly into your bloodstream. A sugar-sweetened beverage can cause a glucose shock in the middle of an otherwise low-glycemic-load meal. So, ironically, even though sugar in liquids has less of an appetite-satisfying effect than sugar in solids, it actually raises blood glucose levels more.

Glucose Shock in a Glass

In the list of glycemic loads in Chapter 4, you probably noticed that the only items with ratings as high as bread, potatoes, and rice are sugar-sweetened beverages and fruit juices. One glass of soda or fruit juice can raise blood glucose levels as high as a serving of starchy food does. A 12-ounce can of Coca-Cola has a glycemic load of 218. An 8-ounce glass of orange juice has a glycemic load of 119. Other fruit juices have even higher ratings.

Pure sugar is overwhelmingly sweet. We tend not to eat much of it unless its sweetness is diluted or disguised—but dilute and disguise is exactly what soft drinks do. They dilute sugar with water and disguise its sweetness with sour ingredients. If drinking a Coke doesn't spoil your appetite, maybe knowing how much sugar is in it will. A 12-ounce can contains *10 teaspoons* of sugar.

Sodas are a major contributor to obesity and diabetes in kids. Although most grown-ups don't drink as much soda (the nondiet kind) as kids do, statistics show that adults who consume even one serving a day double their risk of obesity and diabetes. In one study, women who drank soda daily gained an average of 20 pounds in 9 years and raised their risk of diabetes by 80 percent.

These days, soft drinks are often sweetened with *high-fructose corn syrup,* which contains more of the sugar fructose than cane sugar does. Americans are consuming more fructose than they did 40 years ago, and some nutritionists think this might be playing a role in the obesity epidemic. The usual blood sugar tests do not measure fructose, so glycemic index and load measurements don't take fructose into account. If they did, the glycemic load ratings of soda and fruit drinks would be a lot higher than they are.

If you want to lose weight, you need to kick the soda habit. Fortunately, most grown-ups have little trouble giving up soda. There is one notable exception: folks who have a cola addiction. I've encountered patients who drink 10 to 12 cola drinks a day. Fortunately, these are often sugar-free colas, which suggests that something besides a craving for sugar drives the addiction, most likely an affinity for caffeine. The habit is harmless enough if the beverages are indeed sugar free; however, some cola freaks insist on regular sugar-sweetened cola, repeatedly assailing their bodies with glucose shocks. The best way to deal with this problem is to switch to sugar-free colas. Most cola slaves quickly adjust to the diet versions of their favorite beverages.

When it comes to glucose shocks, sugar-sweetened fruit drinks, including Snapple, SoBe, cranberry juice cocktail, Hawaiian Punch, lemonade, and sports drinks like Gatorade are as bad as, or even worse than, sodas.

Most sugar-free diet drinks are carb free and don't raise blood glucose or insulin levels. However, keep in mind that despite a fivefold per capita increase in diet drink consumption in the last 30 years, the obesity rate has skyrocketed. Some nutritionists think that artificial sweeteners might desensitize people's tastebuds to sweetness and cause them to overeat other sugary foods.

The Facts about Fruit Juice

Fruits in their natural forms are good for you. People who eat lots of fruit have fewer weight problems and a lower incidence of diabetes than people who don't. However, fruit juices, including orange and grapefruit juice, are another story, even if they contain

IN THEIR OWN WORDS

Name and Age: Sheelagh, 60

Pounds Lost: 20 in 3 months

Health Benefits: Reduced insulin need for type 1 diabetes, increased energy

"Restaurants and parties? That's the best part!"

I've had type 1 diabetes for 40 years. My doctor recommended the Glycemic Load Diet, and now, for the first time in my life, I don't feel deprived of food. I have tried all other diets, and the Glycemic Load Diet is the *only* one that works for me. I eat "normal food" now. I have discovered that the more carbs you eat, the more you crave them. You don't need them when you can replace them with all low-glycemic-load foods.

Another benefit? I was surprised by the decrease in the amount of insulin I need, and I have more energy now.

The best part is that I can go to restaurants or parties and not worry about finding something to eat. I love all meat, and I always have a big salad with blue cheese dressing. What could be better than that?

no *added* sugar. Research has linked regular consumption of fruit juice to obesity and diabetes.

Why would fruit in its natural form be good for you but fruit *juice* be harmful? Most of the sugar in a piece of fruit is in the juice. The squeezing process essentially extracts the sugar from several pieces of fruit and puts it all in one serving of juice. Fruit juice is, then, a sugar-sweetened beverage. An 8-ounce glass of orange juice contains the equivalent of 7 teaspoons of sugar.

The juice-making process also removes soluble fiber, which, as I explained in Chapter 5, slows the absorption of sugar. The glycemic load of juice is always higher than that of the intact fruit. In addition, fruit juice, like soda, contains a lot of fructose, which glycemic load measurements don't detect.

Although fruit juice raises blood glucose more than whole fruit does, juice has less of an appetite-satisfying effect. Like other sugar-sweetened beverages, it adds to the calories provided by other foods, rather than replacing them. Orange juice, in particular, is a problem. Although we've been told since we were kids that it's good for us, the truth is, it's a major source of glucose shocks and raises the risk of diabetes and obesity, not to mention tooth decay. My advice is to drink fruit juice only to satisfy a craving for something tangy, never to quench your thirst. If you have to have some juice, don't drink more than 4 ounces—a small glass—at a time.

Alcohol Is Fine, but Beware of Its Appetite-Stimulating Effects

Although beer, wine, and liquor are full of calories, the good news is that they actually don't raise blood glucose levels much. The fermenting process converts most of the sugar in these beverages to alcohol, which provides calories but requires no insulin to metabolize. However, one problem with alcohol is that it blunts sensors in your brain that tell you when you have had enough to eat. A couple of drinks before a meal will make you tend to overeat.

Alcohol can cause you to take in too many calories for another reason: It's addicting. If you're drinking more than one or two alcoholic beverages a day, you're getting enough calories from the drinks themselves to add pounds regardless of their glycemic effects.

"Coffee, Tea, or Milk?"

Before the 1970s, air travelers joked about how often flight attendants had to repeat the question "Coffee, tea, or milk?" Soda and juice weren't among the choices.

Coffee and tea are the most commonly consumed beverages in the world besides water. Scientists have studied them extensively and have never linked them to obesity. In fact, caffeine's stimulant effects encourage weight loss. Recent studies show a reduced incidence of type 2 diabetes among coffee drinkers.

Of course, too much coffee or tea can make you jittery and out of sorts as well as cause insomnia. Also, coffee stimulates stomach acid, which can increase hunger pangs and make you want to eat. Be sure you're not drinking so much as to cause these symptoms.

If you drink only a cup or two of coffee or tea a day, you don't have to worry about adding a little sugar. A teaspoon of table sugar has a glycemic load of 28—not enough to worry about. Artificial sweeteners are fine.

As for milk, Americans are consuming less of it than they did 30 years ago, but the incidence of obesity and diabetes is skyrocketing. Indeed, recent studies show that people who consume generous amounts of dairy products have a *reduced* incidence of obesity and diabetes. The glycemic load of an 8-ounce glass of milk is only 27, making it a great drink for glycemic load watchers.

Water Is Great, but Do We Really Need Eight Glasses a Day?

Only recently in the span of human existence have people had containers to transport water or cups to drink it from. Prehistoric humans had to get down on their hands and knees to sip water from puddles and streams. They didn't drink beverages with every meal. They went for days without any liquids at all.

Nobody knows where the recommendation to drink eight glasses of water a day came from. There are no studies in the medical literature showing any benefit at all from drinking more water than you are naturally inclined to. Indeed, there's plenty of water in fruit, vegetables, meat, and dairy products, not to mention other beverages. Most folks do just fine on a glass or two of liquid a day.

The idea that you should drink more water than you are naturally inclined to probably stems from the notion that it washes toxins out of the body, like running water over a bowl of lettuce to wash away the dirt. In fact, water in excess of what you need to survive doesn't go into the cells of your body. You would die of water toxicity if it did. It goes directly to your kidneys and out in your urine.

Your body has its own powerful mechanisms for regulating water balance. The slightest decrease in your body's water content triggers compelling thirst and an outpouring of the hormone *vasopressin*, which provokes thirst and sharply reduces the amount of water that goes out in your urine. Unless you have a rare vasopressin deficiency, there's no need to try consciously to regulate your fluid intake. Your natural thirst mechanisms do the job just fine.

The simpleminded notion that filling your stomach with water makes you eat less is completely off base. Stretching the stomach with liquids just makes it empty faster and speeds the absorption of glucose. In fact, several things about the way liquids affect digestion suggest that water drinking may actually promote weight gain. Laboratory animals deprived of water sharply curtail their food intake. Beverages consumed with a meal liquefy stomach contents and quicken their entry into the bloodstream. The more liquefied food is, the faster it's digested and the higher it raises blood glucose levels.

My advice is that you make water your thirst quencher of choice (humans are the only animals on Earth that drink anything but water) and let your thirst decide how much you drink.

7

Don't Be Afraid of Sugar

Many people think sugar is some kind of poison, as if a teaspoon or two could expand into pounds of unsightly fat. The truth is, sugar is just another refined carbohydrate. A gram of it won't raise your blood glucose level any higher than a gram of carbohydrate in bread, potatoes, or rice. Ironically, while people seem to feel guilty about eating a few pieces of candy, they think nothing of consuming much more glucose in the form of starch. According to a recent dietary survey, the average American gets more than 20 times more glucose in grain products than in candy. Sweets are not what's making so many of us overweight these days. The problem is starch. Americans don't eat any more candy per capita now than they did before the obesity epidemic began.

Exonerating Sugar

The concept of glycemic load provides another valuable service to humanity: It exonerates sugar. To see how, compare the glycemic indexes of table sugar and peppermint candy with those of white bread and rice. Remember, these are glycemic *indexes*, not loads, so serving size is not specified.

Food	Glycemic Index
White rice	91
Table sugar	97
Peppermint candy	100
White bread	100

This table shows that 50 grams of carbohydrate in white bread or rice will raise your blood sugar as much as 50 grams of carbohydrate in sugar or peppermint candy, but in no way does it exonerate sweets. As far as glycemic *index* (not *load*) is concerned, sugar and candy appear to be just as bad as the starchy items. Now, in the following table, look at the glycemic *loads* (not *indexes*), which adjust for the amounts people typically eat:

Food (serving size)	Glycemic Load
Peppermint candy (1 Life Saver)	20
Table sugar (1 rounded tsp)	28
White bread (1 slice)	100
White rice (1 c)	283

Paints a different picture, doesn't it? Sugar and peppermint candy have much lower glycemic loads than white bread and rice. Why? Simply because *the typical serving sizes are smaller.* Most people don't eat nearly as much table sugar or peppermint candy in a typical serving as they do white bread or rice. This is true of most other candies as long as the sugar in them is not diluted with starch. Consider chocolate. Ounce for ounce, chocolate releases about as much glucose in your bloodstream as a potato does. But how much chocolate can you eat? An amount the size of a potato? If you did, you would get a potato-size glucose shock.

If you're trying to eliminate glucose shocks, a teaspoon of sugar in your coffee, a piece of peppermint candy, or a couple of squares of chocolate won't contribute enough to your glycemic load to cause you trouble. People don't eat large amounts of sugar in solid form, such as in candy, because it's so sweet; you don't need much to satisfy your urge for it.

Unburdening Yourself of Sugar Phobia

It's ironic that we distrust sugar but regard starch as a natural food. We know fruit is good for us, and it contains plenty of sugar. Anthropologists have found evidence that prehistoric humans ate honey, which is 100 percent sugar. Early humans ate fruit and honey for millions of years before starch came on the scene. Our tongues have tastebuds that respond to sugar; we have none that interact with starch.

Paranoia about sugar probably stems from childhood. Sugar was the first food our parents warned us about, but it wasn't because they were worried about our getting fat. It was because they didn't want us to get tooth decay. Indeed, sweets can be bad for children's teeth. However, the problem is not so much candy itself as how many times during the day kids are exposed to it. Acids from the bacterial breakdown of sugar in our mouths erode tooth enamel. Saliva neutralizes those acids and restores enamel, but the neutralization process takes several hours. When kids snack on candy and soda between meals, their saliva doesn't have time to counteract the acids, which eventually promote tooth decay.

Part of people's misconceptions about sugar is a matter of semantics. Doctors have gotten in the habit of calling blood glucose "blood sugar," which leads people to think that the "sugar" in their blood comes from the sugar in sweets. In fact, the sugar in sweets is actually sucrose, a double molecule of glucose and fructose. The sugar in our blood is glucose, which for most of us comes mainly from starch.

Sugar phobia plays into people's fears of obesity and diabetes, but the truth is, a spoonful or two of table sugar or a couple of pieces of candy a day contribute little to glycemic load, as you saw in the example of peppermint candy and white bread. In fact, when it comes to losing weight, sugar can be your ally. Here's how.

Starch Addiction

Although starch is a latecomer to the human diet and we have no biologically natural urge for it, many folks do seem to crave it. In my experience, most overweight people have more difficulty controlling their starch intake than they do their consumption of sweets or fat. That's why a book called *The Carbohydrate Addict's Diet* was a bestseller. What is it about starch that makes people crave it?

When the appetite-regulating centers in your brain want food, they want it fast, and nothing delivers calories into your bloodstream faster than starch. Consequently, we learn to associate starch with immediate satisfaction. We also learn to associate it with tastebud stimulation. "Wait a minute," you're thinking, "didn't you just say that starch is tasteless?" Indeed, it is flavorless. However, saliva contains an enzyme called *amylase* that breaks down a small fraction—about 2 percent—of the starch in your mouth to glucose, which stimulates sweetness receptors on your tongue. The craving for starch, then, is a two-component urge: an impulse to quell hunger fast and a desire for stimulation of tastebuds that sense sweetness.

IN THEIR OWN WORDS

Name and Age: Steve, 59

Pounds Lost: 37 in 12 months

Health Benefits: Lowered cholesterol and triglycerides

"I've lost the weight—and kept it off for more than 3 years!"

I tried low-fat diets several times before, but even though I stuck with them, I just didn't seem to lose weight. This was puzzling because I have always exercised. When I started doing what the book suggested, I went from 213 to 176 pounds in a year and have kept it off for 3 years.

I was amazed that with so little effort, I lost weight steadily. It seemed like I could eat all I wanted. And when I wasn't eating, I wasn't hungry. I don't diet. It's easy.

Going for *Real* Tastebud Stimulation

You can satisfy your urge for starch without actually eating it by addressing the two components of your starch craving separately. The need for quick calories will dissipate if you just give other foods in your meal enough time to satisfy your hunger. If you postpone eating bread, potatoes, or rice until you have finished the rest of your meal, your desire for starch will lessen.

It may not go away, however. Although starch is a lousy tastebud stimulant, chances are the other foods in your meal did not satisfy your sweetness receptors as much as some bread, potatoes, or rice could. Here's the best way to handle the desire for the tastebud stimulation that starch provides: Skip the bread and potatoes and go for the real thing, sugar. Wait until the end of your meal, and then, instead of the starch, have something sweet. That's right—eat dessert. A pinch of sugar will stimulate your tastebuds more than a whole mouthful of starch. You'll find that your urge for starch quickly disappears. You'll finish your meal with your hunger and your desire for tastebud stimulation satisfied.

Keeping Sugar in Its Place

We come by our urge for sweetness naturally. The slight taste of sugar in a plant part let our prehistoric ancestors know that it was probably safe to eat and a source of calories. Although humans ate sugar in pure form in honey for thousands of years before starch came on the scene, you can be sure they didn't eat too much of it. The surly nature of bees saw to that.

Make no mistake, sugar is full of calories, and too much of it can cause your body to overproduce insulin, as any other refined carbohydrate can. It's just that sugar does a better job than starch does of stimulating your tastebuds, curbing your appetite for other foods, and offsetting the calories it adds. Here are some suggestions for making friends with sugar.

- *Avoid "starchy" sweets.* The good news if you have a sweet tooth is that you can enjoy sweets in moderation, as long as they aren't starchy ones. For example, a 1-inch square of

¼-inch-thick dark chocolate has a glycemic load of 39, which is minor. A couple of pieces won't cause a glucose shock. The sugar in chocolate isn't diluted with tasteless starch, so you get to savor every bit of it, which can be tremendously satisfying if you crave something sweet. Other low-starch sweets include jelly beans, peanut brittle, peanut M&Ms, and hard candy.

Cookies, cakes, and pies are another matter. They're full of starch, which passes into your stomach without rousing your tastebuds, requiring you to eat more of it to satisfy your sweet tooth. A typical serving of a baked good releases several times more glucose into your bloodstream than a piece of chocolate does.

- *Use sweets only to stimulate your tastebuds, not to satisfy hunger.* The key to making peace with your sweet tooth is to use sweets only to stimulate your tastebuds, not to satisfy your hunger. Can you eat too much candy? You bet you can. And it's a fact that some sweets taste so good, you tend to overeat them even when you're not hungry. Try to keep in mind that sugar is like nuclear power: It can be a powerful tool, but you have to use it properly. A good rule is to eat only as much as you can wrap the fingers of one hand around.

- *Go sugar free when eating dairy treats.* Sugar-containing dairy products like ice cream, sweetened yogurt, and cheesecake pose a unique problem. Although they contain no starch, they dilute and disguise sugar in the same way soft drinks do. Sugar-sweetened yogurt, cheesecake, and ice cream can give you a glucose shock, whereas no-sugar-added yogurt, cheesecake, and ice cream will not. (Don't make the mistake of confusing *sugar-free* with *low-fat* ice cream or yogurt. These products may have less fat but usually have unacceptable glycemic loads.)

- *Substitute rich, sugarless snacks.* If you want something to munch on and you don't care for sweetness, there are plenty of satisfying sugarless snacks. One of the healthiest is nuts. They are full of protein, fiber, and essential fatty acids, and their glycemic loads are negligible.

Let's face it, if you love sweets, it's foolish to try to live without them. In fact, sugar can make life more pleasurable without necessarily causing harm. Just follow these rules: Avoid starchy sweets, use candy to stimulate your tastebuds and not to satisfy hunger, and don't eat more than a fistful.

8

Activate Your Slow-Twitch Muscles

Maria, age 28, couldn't understand why she had gained 70 pounds in the last 3 years. She didn't think her diet had changed. She worked at a computer all day but had been doing that for several years. The only change in her life was that she had moved to the suburbs and started driving to work instead of walking. Before that, she'd walked a mile to and from work every day. Maria had a hard time believing that walking to work instead of driving was what had kept her from gaining weight.

Bob had gained 50 pounds in 10 years during which he worked as a computer programmer. At age 42, he developed type 2 diabetes. When he reduced his glycemic load and started exercising on weekends, he lost 20 pounds, and his blood glucose measurements improved. However, he found it difficult to lose more weight. Then he had an idea. He started having his wife drop him off 2 miles away from his office so he could walk to work every day. He lost 20 more pounds in a year.

I have often been astonished by the weight-loss benefits of walking to work every day. What is it about regular, low-intensity exercise that relieves insulin resistance so effectively?

You Can Gain without the Pain

It's not your liver, your kidneys, or some other internal organ that causes insulin resistance. It's your muscles. Their lack of responsiveness to insulin makes your pancreas secrete six to eight times the normal amounts of the hormone to handle the carbohydrates you eat. The good news is that you can restore your muscles' sensitivity to insulin. You do it with exercise, but not the kind you're probably thinking of, not the sweaty, exhausting kind. When it comes to reversing insulin resistance, the benefits of exercise don't necessarily correlate with strenuousness.

Let me illustrate this with a true story. A group of researchers in Switzerland worked in a clinic near a mountain. There were two ways to get to the top—you could traverse a 2-mile path or ride a tram. The scientists decided to compare the effects on blood sugar of walking up the mountain and riding the tram down versus taking the tram up and walking down. After 2 months, they measured their subjects' responses to a glucose load. To the researchers' surprise, walking downhill improved insulin sensitivity more than walking uphill did.

The point is that the no-pain, no-gain philosophy of exercise doesn't always apply. Certainly, if you're training for a footrace or trying to build big muscles, you need to sweat and strain, and walking uphill would be better than walking down. However, some kinds of muscle activity create less fatigue than others do, and if you're trying to relieve insulin resistance, it so happens that the less fatiguing kind is exactly the kind you need. To understand how this is so, you need to consider what causes insulin resistance.

The Genetic Defect Underlying Insulin Resistance

Researchers have recently pinpointed the biochemical quirk that causes some people's muscles to lose sensitivity to insulin when they don't exercise enough. It's a genetic defect in the tiny energy-producing units of muscles called *mitochondria*. These little dynamos use oxygen to burn glucose and fat and produce the energy that powers muscles.

The difference between people who are genetically prone to developing insulin resistance and those who are not is that the mitochondria of those predisposed to insulin resistance go into a deeper-than-normal dormant state when they haven't been used. It's like my computer. If I don't use it for an hour, it automatically goes into "sleep mode." It's not completely shut off; parts of it are still running, and if I press a key, it immediately starts up again. But while it's in the sleep mode, it uses less energy.

That's the way your muscles respond to exercise if you have insulin resistance. If you don't use them for a day or two, they go into a kind of sleep mode in which they burn fewer calories and stop responding to insulin. When you exercise them again, they quickly wake up. They remain sensitive to insulin for 24 to 48 hours, and then they shut back down.

The message should be clear. If you keep your muscles from going into sleep mode—by exercising them every 24 to 48 hours—they will maintain their sensitivity to insulin, your pancreas won't have to make as much insulin, and your body will stop trying to store calories as fat.

Muscles That Don't Fatigue

To understand how it's possible to keep your metabolism humming like a long-distance runner's without a lot of huffing or puffing, you need to know about the two different kinds of muscle fibers in your body. Your muscles comprise a mix of two different types of muscle fibers. One kind contracts slower than the other does, so they're called "slow-twitch" fibers. The others are "fast-twitch" fibers. Each type specializes in its own kind of exercise. Slow-twitch fibers provide power for steady, long-distance activities like walking or jogging. You use fast-twitch fibers for short bursts of intense effort like weight lifting or sprinting. The important difference between the two kinds of muscle fibers is that slow-twitch fibers require oxygen to do their work, and fast-twitch fibers do not—at least not immediately. They go into "oxygen debt," replenishing their energy after their work is completed.

Because slow-twitch fibers need more oxygen while they're working than fast-twitch fibers do, they have more mitochondria, which, as you recall, is exactly where the problem is if you have insulin resistance. That's why exercise like walking or jogging, which depends on slow-twitch fibers, reduces insulin resistance and promotes weight loss better than short bursts of more strenuous exertion like weight lifting, which use mainly fast-twitch fibers.

Now, you may find it hard to believe that you can lose weight without strenuous exertion, but think for a moment about your diaphragm, the muscle under your rib cage that moves air in and out of your lungs. How much effort does it take to exercise that muscle to breathe? You're not even aware you're doing it. It's a fact: Certain muscles can work steadily for long periods without causing fatigue. The reason such muscles can operate without producing a sense of tiredness is that they're powered by slow-twitch muscle fibers. As slow-twitch fibers work, oxygen constantly replenishes their energy.

A light should have just come on in your brain: Slow-twitch fibers are where the problem is if you have insulin resistance. How convenient! The kind of exercise you need to restore your body's sensitivity to insulin is exactly the kind that requires the least effort. You don't need to sweat and strain to lose weight. All you have to do is turn on those oxygen-burning mitochondria in your slow-twitch muscle fibers. Here's how to do it.

Keeping Your Slow-Twitch Fibers Out of "Sleep Mode"

Because all animals need to breathe and get from one place to another, Mother Nature made sure that the muscles that perform those tasks operate with as little effort as possible. Consequently, those activities rely almost entirely on slow-twitch muscle fibers. Of course, your breathing muscles are only a small part of your total muscle mass, so they contribute little to your metabolism. But the muscles that propel you, your walking muscles, are a different story. They represent about 70 percent of your muscle mass. Activating them has a profound effect on your body chemistry.

And that's where the problem lies: Modern humans are the only creatures in the history of the world that don't depend on muscle power to get from one place to another. Although a change in dietary habits triggered the rise in obesity of the last 40 years, the stage was set by the marked reduction in muscle activity that occurred over the previous century as engines took over the task of moving us from one place to another. Think about how little we modern folks walk compared with our ancestors. Prehistoric humans spent most of their waking hours scrambling across rugged terrain in search of food and game. They migrated hundreds of miles as the seasons changed. As recently as the early 1900s, people thought nothing of walking 4 or 5 miles a day to get to and from their jobs and spent most of their workday on their feet. Now it's a big deal if you have to walk across a parking lot or up a flight of stairs. We use our walking muscles a pitiful fraction of the amount our ancestors did.

Considering that most of the mitochondria in our bodies reside in our walking muscles, it's not surprising that so many of us are insulin resistant. The reason our metabolisms are out of whack is not that we don't go to health clubs, lift weights, or run marathons. It's because we don't walk. We don't use our slow-twitch muscle fibers enough to keep them out of sleep mode.

The Optimal Oxygen-Burning Pace

Our ancestors walked simply to get from point A to point B. They weren't doing it to keep in shape. They didn't have to push themselves; you don't have to push yourself either. The next time you go for a walk, pay attention to how much effort you're expending. If you walk fast enough, you become air-hungry, and your legs start to feel tired. If you're not an exercise lover, you might describe that as strenuous. But notice what happens when you decrease your walking speed just a little. You will find that you don't have to slow down much before the shortness of breath and leg fatigue abruptly stop. You quickly reach a point where you don't sense you're expending much effort at all. What's happening? That's the level of exertion at which the energy you expend powering your slow-twitch muscle fibers is being completely replenished by oxygen. You aren't pushing your muscles beyond their capacity, and you're not building up an oxygen debt by enlisting your fast-twitch fibers. You stop thinking about how hard you're working, and your mind moves on to other things. At that pace, you feel as if you could walk indefinitely. You might be bored, you might be in a hurry to get home, but you cannot honestly say that what you're doing is strenuous. That's all the harder you need to work to relieve insulin resistance and lose weight.

Make no mistake, there are benefits to more strenuous exercise—you can build more endurance and develop stronger muscles. But remember what you're trying to accomplish. You're not training for a footrace or trying to build big muscles. You're just trying to restore your muscles' sensitivity to insulin, and happily, there's a disconnect between strenuousness of exercise and its effectiveness for reversing insulin resistance. You don't have to push yourself. All you have to do is take yourself back to earlier times when obesity and diabetes were rare and use your leg muscles as nature intended, to walk at a comfortable pace.

Turning On Your Metabolic "Switch"

If it's inconvenient to walk—if the weather's bad or if you can't find a place to do it—you can activate your slow-twitch muscle fibers with a StairMaster, elliptical trainer, or stationary bike. For easiness, however, there's nothing better than walking. Exercise physiologists have found that, of all the different kinds of exercise, walking burns the most calories with the least perceived effort. In other words, you might not think you're exercising much when you're walking, but you really are. Study after study proves that for losing weight and preventing diabetes, walking is just as effective as running or working out at a gym.

Although walking is all you need to do to activate the biochemical pathways in your muscles that allow them to respond to insulin, you can't get these reactions going by sauntering over to the watercooler. You need to walk farther than that. However, insulin sensitivity exhibits a sort of all-or-none phenomenon—like a switch, it's either on or off. Once you do enough exercise to get those metabolic processes started—in other words, once you turn on the switch—you don't need to do much more. You've already learned that you don't have to engage in strenuous exercise to activate your slow-twitch fibers; walking at a comfortable pace is just fine. So how much walking do you need to do to switch on your insulin sensitivity?

Scientists have found that it takes between 20 and 30 minutes of walking to switch on insulin sensitivity. Exercising more than that might be good for other things—you might burn more calories or get in better shape—but it's unnecessary if you're just trying to lose weight.

Research studies show that the weight-loss benefit of going from getting no regular exercise to walking just 20 minutes every other day is actually greater than the benefit of going from walking regularly to being a long-distance runner. The point is not just that exercise is good for you—you already knew that—but that getting no exercise is *terrible* for you.

Nevertheless, as long as you're out there walking, you might want to do enough to guarantee that you shed pounds. Most studies show that people consistently lose weight—even if they don't change their diet—if they walk 40 minutes four times a week. That's about 2 miles every other day.

The 48-Hour Rule

When it comes to losing weight, the frequency of exercise is more important than the intensity. Whatever kind of exercise you do, you need to do it at least every other day. It doesn't matter if you walk a couple of miles or run a marathon. About 48 hours later, your muscles stop responding to insulin. Exercising only on weekends, even if it's very vigorous, won't do the job. Considering that the beneficial effects of exercise last only 48 hours, if you have a sedentary job and exercise only on weekends, your body spends 4 days a week in a state of insulin resistance. This means for 4 days out of 7, you have higher-than-normal insulin levels, your weight-regulating systems are out of kilter, and your body tries to store calories as fat.

Relatively sedentary activities like walking around an office, retrieving files, or doing light housework are no substitute for aerobic exercise, but if such movements are performed hundreds of times a day, they contribute significantly to energy expenditure. Conversely, the fewer such movements you make throughout the day, the greater your tendency to gain weight. Researchers call this the *fidget factor,* and it significantly influences your ability to lose weight.

Two common activities have very low fidget factors: working on a computer and watching television. Observe someone doing these things. He or she hardly moves a muscle for several minutes at a time. Television screens and computer monitors seem to mesmerize people, freezing their body movements. Some of the worst physically conditioned people I see in my medical practice are computer workers. If you spend more than 8 hours a day in front of a computer or television screen, walking every other day might not be enough. You probably need to exercise daily.

Enhancing the Pleasure and Comfort of Walking

Chances are you'll enjoy walking for its own sake. It provides a respite from day-to-day hassles, gives you some time to gather your thoughts, and puts you in touch with the physical world. Regular walking stimulates the body's natural antidepressant

---

IN THEIR OWN WORDS

Name and Age: Shannon, 37

Pounds Lost: 20 in 3 months

Health Benefits: Increased energy, decreased blood sugar fluctuations, lost 10 inches from waist

"I got my waist back!"

A friend of mine gave me a copy of The Glycemic Load Diet. After doing what the book said for 3 months, I lost 20 pounds. What amazed me, though, was what happened to my waistline. It shrank 10 inches!

I've tried Atkins, Weight Watchers, and other diets. This is the easiest to stay on. I worry less about what I am going to eat. I don't have too many restrictions. There are always options other than bread, rice, and pasta. It's so easy to follow.

hormones and is actually as effective as medication for relieving mild depression.

However, if walking isn't entertaining enough for you, modern technology can help. A portable CD or MP3 player will allow you to listen to music, lectures, or audio versions of books as you walk. One devoted hoofer told me she gets so engaged listening to audiobooks that she often extends her route so she can listen longer.

If you're starting a walking program for the first time, I suggest you buy a couple of heel pads at your local drugstore and wear them for a month or two as your feet toughen up. The most common cause of persistent foot pain upon starting a walking program is something called *plantar fasciitis,* which causes painful heels. The pads will help prevent that.

If walking makes the balls of your feet or your big toe joints hurt, try a pair of cheap arch supports, which you can buy at most drugstores. They redistribute the pressure on your feet and help prevent soreness.

Beyond Walking: The Role of Resistance Exercise

Your muscles are the main fuel consumers of your body and the target of most of the insulin you produce. The more muscle tissue you have, the easier it is to burn calories and the more sensitive you are to insulin. If you are already walking or jogging enough to switch on your insulin sensitivity and you want to rev up your metabolism further, work to increase your muscle mass. The best way to do that is through *resistance* exercise, straining your muscles against resistance.

The beauty of *resistance* exercise is that it has to be done for only a few minutes per week to build and maintain muscle mass, as long as effort is expended against maximum resistance. The following twice-a-week, 15-minute routine is possible to do quickly at the gym or at home and has been proven by exercise physiologists to do the job. For each muscle group, do two sets of 10 repetitions, the first set using 80 percent of the maximum weight you can lift 10 times, and the second set using 100 percent of the maximum weight you can lift 10 times.

Three exercises for the arms:

Biceps curl: Grip a dumbbell in each hand. Keeping your upper arms close to your sides, bend your elbows to curl your palms toward your shoulders. Lower and repeat.

Triceps press: Sit on a bench or stand holding a barbell straight over your head with your back straight. Lower the bar down behind your neck in an arc, keeping your elbows stationary. Now press the bar upward and get a full triceps extension.

Shoulder lift: Stand with your feet together and arms at your sides, holding a dumbbell in each hand. Keeping your elbows slightly bent, raise your arms out to the sides, palms down. When they're at about shoulder height, bend your elbows 90 degrees so your forearms are vertical and palms face forward. Then press the dumbbells straight up overhead. Slowly reverse back to the starting position.

Three exercises for the legs:

Knee extension: Start with your back against a wall, with your right leg bent and foot flat on the floor. Extend your left leg straight out in front of you, about 8 inches above the floor. Bring your left leg in and extend it back out straight with your toes up. Switch legs and repeat.

Hamstring curl: Lie facedown on the floor. Bending your left knee, bring your foot toward your butt until your leg is bent at a 90-degree angle. Keep your hips on the floor and your foot flexed. Slowly lower your foot. Repeat with your right leg.

Squat: Stand with your back to a chair. Bending at the knees and hips, lower yourself as though you're sitting down. Keep your back straight and make sure you can always see your toes. Stop just shy of touching the chair, then stand back up.

Most gyms have equipment designed for this kind of exercise, but you can get a similar workout with a pair of heavy dumbbells.

If you're worried that you might become *too* muscular, relax. After age 30, it's almost impossible to develop bulky muscles. You'll just look more fit.

Remember: Weight loss tends to slow your metabolism, but exercise revs it up—and not just while you're doing it, but 24 hours a day. Weight lifting works by preserving muscle mass. Aerobic exercise like walking or jogging works by increasing the size and number of mitochondria in your slow-twitch muscles and enhancing your body's sensitivity to insulin. Researchers have found that the main difference between people who develop weight problems as they age and those who don't is not so much their diet as their exercise level. So put on your walking shoes and hit the pavement.

There's only one good thing about being overweight: You have great leg muscles. Get those babies moving, and they'll do wonders for your metabolism. If you add 40 minutes of slow-twitch muscle activation every other day to a low-glycemic-load diet, your body will work much differently than it did before. Your insulin levels will drop like a rock, your triglyceride level will plummet, and your body's natural antidepressant hormones will surge. Immediately, you'll feel better, and soon you'll start looking better.

9

Avoiding Diet-Induced Metabolic Slowdown

None of us wants to deprive ourselves of the enjoyment of food. We'll go on a diet, but we want it to be over as soon as possible. We approach weight loss with a fix-it mentality. We want to get the job done and return to business as usual as quickly as possible. Our usual strategy, then, is to put ourselves through a period of deprivation until we reach a goal and then to go back to our old ways, with minor modifications to maintain weight loss. At least that's the plan—and that's the problem.

Without a doubt, the greatest obstacle to successful weight loss is the concept of "dieting," the idea of putting yourself through a period of deprivation that ends when the goal is reached. As rational as that strategy might seem—and we persist in trying it over and over again—it virtually guarantees failure.

Crash Dieting: A Metabolic Train Wreck

Most doctors, nutritionists, and diet book authors know that rapid-weight-loss diets usually fail. People shed pounds initially but usually gain them back plus more. Why, then, do they persist in recommending this approach? Because it's what people expect.

Two popular low-carb diets, the Atkins Diet and the South Beach Diet, recommend kicking off their regimens with a period of strict carbohydrate restriction called the "induction phase." Purportedly, the idea is to purge dieters' carbohydrate cravings— like putting an alcoholic in a detox ward to get him off booze. This near-total carbohydrate restriction causes substantial weight loss in just a week or two. Although much of that is water loss and not true fat depletion, its real purpose is to boost dieters' morale and give them an incentive to continue. It also inspires them to spread the word of how effective their latest diet is.

Call these regimens what you will, but they're crash diets, the same old strategy of starving weight off with a strict diet not intended to be maintained indefinitely. This approach to weight loss contains the seeds of its own destruction. Here's why.

Crash dieting of any kind—whether low carb or low fat— throws your body chemistry into a sort of starvation mode. Within a few days, your metabolism starts to fight back. Powerful hormonal reactions slow your metabolism to prevent weight loss. This slowdown deepens over the course of weeks, making it increasingly difficult to lose weight. But here's the really bad news: Diet-induced metabolic slowdown doesn't go away when you stop dieting. It continues after you return to normal eating, making it almost inevitable that you gain back the weight you lost. The worst of it is, this starvation mode persists *after* you regain the weight you've lost, encouraging you to gain even more weight. Alas, most crash diets result in weight gain, not loss. The word *crash* is appropriate: It's a metabolic train wreck!

Crash diets and induction phases are wrong for another reason. They restrict nutritious foods. After a week or two, dieters start craving what they're missing. These cravings, combined with diet-induced metabolic slowdown, practically guarantee failure.

The Ketosis Myth

Atkins and others in his time were impressed with a phenomenon called *ketosis*. If you eliminate all carbohydrates, after several hours your body starts converting fat and protein to glucose. This process produces natural chemical by-products called *ketones*. Some of these substances end up in your urine and can be detected with a simple chemical test.

Atkins advocated restricting carbs until ketones appeared in the urine. He thought this meant that people were literally flushing calories down the drain—an attractive notion, indeed, but one that has since been disproved. The number of calories you lose this way is inconsequential. Researchers have put subjects on low-glycemic-load diets with enough carbohydrates in fruits and vegetables to prevent ketosis and have found little difference in weight loss from that produced by near-total carbohydrate restriction.

A Role for Resistance Exercise

As crucial as moderate, continuous exercise like walking or jogging is for improving insulin sensitivity and shedding pounds, resistance exercise such as weight lifting has a special role when it comes to losing weight. It prevents the metabolic slowdown that accompanies rapid weight loss. Strict diets cause muscles to shrink, which reduces the number of calories they burn during exercise and rest and contributes heavily to diet-induced metabolic slowdown.

Resistance exercise is superior to other kinds of exercise for building and maintaining muscle mass. If you find that you are losing weight fast—say, more than 7 pounds the first month or 4 pounds a month thereafter—it's a good idea to add some resistance exercises, such as the program suggested in Chapter 8, to your aerobic program.

The Rapid-Weight-Loss Fairy Tale

You've seen the ads suggesting you can diet away 30 or 40 pounds in a few weeks. The truth is, that kind of weight loss is usually a combination of dehydration, muscle shrinkage, inaccurate measurement, and self-delusion. If you came anywhere near losing that much fat that fast, you would shut down your metabolism for years. Rapid weight loss invariably sets you up for equally rapid weight gain.

How much weight loss can you reasonably expect? Cutting out starch and sugar typically causes about 3 pounds of water loss and 2 pounds of fat loss the first month. Walking 2 miles every other day burns off another 2 pounds. That makes 7 pounds the first month and 4 pounds per month thereafter. And that's enough! If you lose more than that, you risk shutting down your metabolism.

Heading Off Metabolic Slowdown Before It Hits

Scientists can detect metabolic slowdown within a few days of a subject's starting a strict diet. Some slowing probably occurs within a few hours, which would suggest that it's important not to skip meals. While scientists have not yet discovered the internal signal that triggers diet-induced metabolic slowing, undoubtedly a sense of hunger accompanies it. To keep your body chemistry humming, you need to keep the metabolic furnaces stoked. You should answer the call of hunger. The good news is that low-glycemic-load diets cause less metabolic slowing than low-fat diets do. Making a point of including fat and protein in your diet helps avoid diet-induced metabolic slowdown.

Unless you visit a research laboratory every day, it's impossible to tell if your body chemistry is slowing down. The best strategy is to prevent diet-induced metabolic slowdown before it occurs. Here are some suggestions.

- Rid yourself of the "dieting" mentality. Make modest changes you can stick with permanently.
- Avoid rapid weight loss (more than 7 pounds the first month or 4 pounds a month thereafter).
- Do not try to lose weight by reducing food intake alone. *Always* add aerobic exercise like walking or jogging.
- Maintain adequate fat intake.
- Don't skip meals.
- Add resistance exercise if you find yourself losing more than 3 or 4 pounds a month.

If you lose only a couple of pounds a month but you're comfortable doing it, your confidence will return. You will see that losing weight is easier than you thought, and you'll know you've found a healthier way of living you can continue for life.

Part 3

Eating the
Low-Glycemic-
Load Way

10

Getting a Healthy Mix of Fats

To lose weight, the only thing you need to know about fat is that it adds calories. However, the food we eat contains several kinds of fat, and each type plays a unique role in our body chemistries. Scientists are not yet sure of the importance of these differences among fats, but they know that humans lived for millions of years on diets with a particular balance among the various kinds. Indeed, a change in the balance of fats in your diet can influence your good and bad cholesterol levels. Although these effects are usually modest—not nearly as important as genetics—they're worth knowing about. Remember, though, for you to lose weight, your top priority must be to eliminate refined carbohydrates. My advice is not to try to reduce your intake of any kind of fat; the wider the variety of foods you have to choose from, the easier it will be to cut starch and sugar. What you should do, however, is make sure you're eating a healthy *mix* of fats. To do that, you need to know about the different kinds of fats.

Saturated and Unsaturated Fats

The first distinction you should make is between saturated and unsaturated fat. You can actually tell the difference just by looking at them. Saturated fats are solid at room temperature; an example is the rind of fat (the suet) that surrounds a steak. Unsaturated fats are liquid at room temperature; an example is olive oil.

Most of the saturated fat we eat comes from the visible fat in meat and the fat in milk products (the butterfat). We get unsaturated fat also from meat and dairy products and from oily plant foods like nuts, soybeans, olives, and avocados.

The reason it's important to distinguish between saturated and unsaturated fat is that they have slightly different effects on the levels of cholesterol in your blood. Remember that most heart attack patients do *not* have particularly high blood cholesterol levels. More often, they have low levels of good cholesterol, HDL, a type of particle in your blood that removes cholesterol from arteries.

Although saturated fats tend to raise bad cholesterol levels, they also raise good cholesterol. Unsaturated fats tend to lower bad cholesterol a little and raise good cholesterol. So if you reduce your intake of saturated fats and increase your consumption of unsaturated fats, your bad cholesterol level will usually decline modestly, on average between 5 and 10 percent, and your HDL level will stay the same or increase slightly. However, results vary. Your bad cholesterol might fall more or not at all. Often it goes down initially and then comes back up after a few months.

Reducing saturated fats alone—without increasing unsaturated fats—does little to your bad cholesterol levels and tends to lower good cholesterol. In the Dietary Modification Arm of the Women's Health Initiative, dietitians gave intensive low-fat, low-cholesterol diet counseling to 18,000 women but made no attempt to increase their intake of unsaturated fat. After 8 years, bad cholesterol levels fell less than 2 percent, and there was no effect on the incidence of heart disease.

One problem with trying to reduce fat in your diet—other than depriving you of some of your favorite foods and encouraging you to eat more starch—is that it tends to lower the blood levels of good cholesterol. Indeed, a good way to raise your good cholesterol level is to eat less carbohydrate and *more* fat.

For years, scientists have been trying to develop good medications to raise HDL levels, but the only pills that work often have intolerable side effects. Recent diet studies show that reducing carbs and eating more fat raises HDL a little—about 5 percent. Similarly, doctors have known for years that regular exercise raises HDL levels a little—again, about 5 percent. However, if you do both—exercise regularly *and* reduce carbs—bingo! You get a big jump in your good cholesterol level. In 2010, the *Annals of Internal Medicine* reported the results of a study of 307 overweight subjects, half of whom were instructed to follow a low-glycemic-load, liberalized fat diet and walk 50 minutes, 5 days a week. The other half were told to follow a low-fat, low-calorie diet and given no instructions to exercise. In those who cut carbs and walked regularly, HDL increased 23 percent, as large an increase as you can get from taking any medication available.

Mono- versus Polyunsaturated Oils

Scientists divide the oils (unsaturated fat) we eat into two categories: monounsaturated and polyunsaturated. Because both are oils, you can't tell the difference just by looking at them.

Monounsaturated fats are somewhat hard to come by in our diet. We get them mainly from certain oily plant foods—namely, olives, nuts, and avocados. Polyunsaturated fats are more abundant. Vegetable oils, including corn, soybean, and peanut oil, as well as meat and fish contain plenty of polyunsaturated fats.

Monounsaturated fats actually lower bad cholesterol slightly and raise good cholesterol. Many nutritionists believe that these fats are good for the heart and blood vessels. Inhabitants of some countries where olive oil provides a large portion of the fat eaten have a lower incidence of heart disease than do people from parts of the world where olive oil is not such a large part of the diet. However, other factors may explain those differences.

Polyunsaturated fats also lower bad cholesterol levels a little, but they lower good cholesterol, too. Their net effect, although probably not harmful, is likely not beneficial either.

If you find it hard to keep track of the different kinds of fats, a good rule of thumb is to try to get as much fat from vegetable products such as olive oil, avocados, and nuts as you do from animal sources.

Getting Your Omega-3 Fatty Acids

When your body needs a particular type of fat, it can usually convert other kinds to whatever type it requires. However, there are a few fats your system can't manufacture, so you have to rely on dietary intake to provide them. Because it's essential that you get these fats in your food, they're called *essential* fatty acids. Your body uses them to make cell membranes, hormones, and other important things.

The hardest kind of essential fatty acid to come by is a type of polyunsaturated fat called *omega-3* fatty acid. Humans aren't alone in being unable to manufacture omega-3s. No member of the animal kingdom can. Only certain plants synthesize them, mainly leaves, grasses, and algae. Because we don't eat these kinds of plants, we get most of our essential fatty acids from the meat of animals that do, including grass-eating animals such as cattle and sheep, and fish that consume smaller algae-eating creatures.

In the past, we got enough omega-3s in the meat we ate. However, these days, instead of allowing cows and sheep to graze on natural foliage, ranchers confine them to feedlots and fatten them up with grain, which contains little omega-3 fatty acid. As a result, our diets are becoming increasingly deficient in this nutrient. Although no common diseases are known to be caused by omega-3 deficiency, there is no doubt that we modern humans are eating less than our ancestors did. Many experts believe that supplementing the diet with omega-3s has beneficial effects on the heart and blood vessels as well as several other systems in the body.

The best source of omega-3 fatty acids is certain cold-water fish, including salmon and sardines. Walnuts and flaxseed oil also are good sources. Fish oil capsules or a handful of walnuts a day or two servings of cold-water fish a week, which is what the American Heart Association recommends, should ensure adequate intake.

The Trans Fat Controversy

Polyunsaturated fat becomes rancid after a few days of exposure to air at room temperature, which limits the shelf life of food that contains it. Food manufacturers learned to get around this problem by using a process called *partial hydrogenation,* heating the oil for several hours in the presence of hydrogen gas. Partial hydrogenation extends the shelf life of baked goods and margarines made with vegetable oil. If you look at the labels on packages of cookies, crackers, chips, or margarine, you'll usually find the phrase "partially hydrogenated oil."

In the 1970s, after food scientists discovered that polyunsaturated fat lowered cholesterol a little or at least did not raise it, they began recommending that people consume more unsaturated fat and less saturated fat. For years, folks thought they were doing themselves a favor by eating products made from polyunsaturated fats instead of butterfat and lard, and the food industry changed to accommodate this preference. Then, in the 1990s, scientists discovered a problem. The high temperatures used during partial hydrogenation damaged polyunsaturated fat, changing some of it to an unnatural kind of fat called *trans fat.* It turns out that trans fat raises blood cholesterol levels as much as butter and lard do, but unlike saturated fat, it lowers good cholesterol. Some scientists believe that trans fat is more harmful than any of the other kinds of fats. Some cities have passed laws prohibiting its use in food preparation.

Medical science isn't yet sure what kinds of problems trans fat can cause, but doctors are suspicious of it. The American Heart Association still recommends unsaturated over saturated fat but suggests limiting consumption of margarines and partially hydrogenated oils until scientists learn more about them.

Here's the good news: If you reduce your glycemic load, you don't have to worry a bit about trans fat. That's because cutting out refined carbohydrates gets rid of the shortening, cooking oil and margarine you consume to make starch palatable. The fact is that most of the partially hydrogenated fat in our diet is in the starch we eat. When you cut out commercially prepared cookies, crackers, and chips, you get rid of the partially hydrogenated oils that go with them, and when you eliminate bread, potatoes, and rice, you no longer need margarine to make them taste better.

Putting Fat in Perspective

Atkins proved to the world that people can eat fatty foods and still lose weight. You might ask, then, why you would want to pay attention to your fat intake. Here's the best reason: Not going overboard on fat makes room in your diet for fruits, vegetables, and sweets, and it's the lack of those foods that foils most people's attempts to stay on a low-carb diet.

The good news is, if you eliminate starch, you usually don't have to consciously avoid fat. That's because cutting out refined carbohydrates gets rid of the shortening, cooking oil, margarine, gravy, cream cheese, and butter you consume to make starch palatable. You experience a pleasant paradox: You can eat more meat, dairy products, nuts, and olives than you did before without actually increasing your fat consumption. It might seem like you're eating more fat, but you're really not. Research studies have shown repeatedly that people on low-carb diets who eat all the eggs, meat, dairy products, and fatty vegetable products they want end up consuming fewer calories on average than people on low-fat diets who consciously try to cut calories, and they tend *not* to overeat fat. Certainly, you don't need to try to eat more fat than you normally would. It's the reduced starch, not the liberalized fat, that makes people lose weight on low-carb diets. I suggest you limit yourself to average American serving sizes of meat and dairy products, with a half-portion second helping if you wish. (Typical serving sizes are listed in Appendix A.) In addition, here are some suggestions for attaining a natural balance among the fats in your diet.

- Cut away the visible fat in meat, preferably before cooking.
- Choose lean hamburger. Better yet, pick a lean cut of sirloin and ask your butcher to grind it for you.
- Eat several helpings of nuts, olives, or avocados weekly.
- Whenever possible, use olive oil—preferably high-quality extra virgin olive oil—in place of other kinds of oils, margarine, and butter.
- Eat at least one serving of salmon, trout, sardines, herring, or mackerel weekly.
- Consider taking a fish oil supplement.

Remember, if worrying about the kinds of fats in your diet reduces the enjoyment you get from your low-glycemic-load eating style and causes you to eat more starch, it's not worth the trouble. Make no mistake, the benefits of optimizing your fat balance are largely theoretical and are dwarfed by the advantages of losing weight by any means. Any changes suggested in this chapter are worth making only if you're sure they won't interfere with your weight-loss program.

11

Managing Cholesterol with a Low-Glycemic-Load Diet

Bill not only had high blood cholesterol but was 35 pounds overweight and had signs of insulin resistance. To lower his cholesterol, he tried cutting out eggs, meat, and dairy products but found himself eating more starch and sugar. Although his cholesterol level dropped a few points, it was still too high, and he gained 10 more pounds.

Then his doctor prescribed cholesterol-lowering medication. One pill a day lowered his cholesterol level to normal and allowed him to go back to eating eggs, meat, and dairy products. He was then able to focus his efforts on reducing starch and sugar in his diet and relieving insulin resistance. He found it easier to lose weight, and his cholesterol level was lower than ever.

Bill typifies many patients who try to lower their blood cholesterol by going on low-cholesterol diets. They don't succeed in lowering their cholesterol levels enough to reduce their risk of heart disease much; they just end up eating more starch and sugar. Bill succeeded in lowering his cholesterol level *and* losing weight when he approached the cholesterol and carbohydrate parts of his metabolism separately. He used medication to reduce his cholesterol level and devoted his dietary efforts to improving his carbohydrate metabolism.

Rethinking Cholesterol

It was no coincidence that shortly after government agencies and medical organizations started warning the public about dietary cholesterol, the obesity rate suddenly shot up. Cholesterol fears triggered a shift in eating patterns away from eggs, meat, and dairy products toward more flour products, potatoes, and rice. Forty years later, the lesson medical science learned—or should have learned—is that making people afraid to eat cholesterol doesn't do much to prevent heart disease but dramatically increases the risk of obesity and diabetes.

If you want to lose weight, you need to purge your thinking of the anticholesterol propaganda you've been exposed to for the past 40 years. It's not that reducing cholesterol is of itself bad. The problem is, you have to eat something, and as a practical matter, if you can't eat eggs, meat, and dairy products, you're probably going to eat more refined carbohydrates.

Is cholesterol important? You bet it is. Infiltration of arteries by cholesterol is the leading cause of death and disability of Americans and Europeans. Reducing cholesterol levels in the blood prevents heart disease more effectively than any other treatment known. The problem is that reducing cholesterol in your food does little to reduce the cholesterol in your blood. Your body makes its own cholesterol. It manufactures about three times more than you eat. If you eat less, it just makes more. Moreover, your digestive system absorbs only about half of the cholesterol in your food. Most of it goes out in your stool. The level of cholesterol in your blood depends mainly on how efficient your system is at removing it, not on how much cholesterol you eat. High blood cholesterol is caused by genetic deficiencies of cellular receptors responsible for removing cholesterol particles from your blood, and has little to do with your diet.

Where, then, did we get the notion that dietary cholesterol causes heart disease? It sounds reasonable. You are what you eat, right? And, in one sense, it's true: People who live in certain parts of the world where starvation is a constant threat have lower blood cholesterol levels and fewer heart attacks than inhabitants of wealthier countries do. But short of such deprivation, reducing *dietary* cholesterol has little effect on *blood* cholesterol. Closely supervised low-fat, low-cholesterol diets reduce blood cholesterol levels between 5 and 10 percent at best, which is not enough to make much of a dent in your risk of heart disease.

Two Separate Parts of Your Body Chemistry

The cholesterol side of your metabolism is largely independent of the carbohydrate side. While your cholesterol level is determined mainly by your genes and has little to do with your diet and exercise habits, how well your body handles carbohydrates is *strongly* influenced by diet and exercise. In other words, your genes control the cholesterol side; your lifestyle governs the carbohydrate side.

Things that are good for the cholesterol side of your metabolism aren't necessarily good for the carbohydrate side. For example, eating less meat and fewer eggs and dairy products might lower your bad cholesterol level a little, but if it causes you to eat more starch and sugar, it will aggravate insulin resistance and encourage weight gain. Conversely, cutting carbs might help you lose weight but might not lower bad cholesterol. To achieve a good metabolic balance, you need to manage the cholesterol and the carbohydrate parts of your body chemistry separately.

Doing Right by Your Arteries

Once you understand how high blood cholesterol causes heart attacks, you will see clearly what you need to do to keep your arteries healthy. A heart attack occurs when an artery to the heart muscle is suddenly blocked off. Contrary to common belief, cholesterol doesn't steadily build up in arteries until they become blocked. When too many cholesterol particles start accumulating in artery walls, the body fights back. Defensive cells called *macrophages* attack cholesterol particles as if they were foreign invaders like bacteria or viruses. Normally, when macrophages encounter bacteria or viruses, they secrete some nasty enzymes called *proteinases*, which kill the intruders. Although proteinases are good for killing germs, they don't do much to cholesterol. But that doesn't deter the macrophages; they keep secreting their enzymes anyway, and that's the problem. If the battle gets intense enough, the enzymes start burning cavities in the artery wall. These cavities fill with a pasty mix of cholesterol and dead macrophages, creating soft pockets that lie under the inner lining of arteries like boils under the skin.

These "boils" are what cause heart attacks. Like boils, they sometimes burst and rip the inner lining of the artery. The body then tries to repair the tear by forming a blood clot over it. Here's where the body makes a mistake: Sometimes the clot gets so big it blocks the artery and cuts off bloodflow to the heart muscle.

Now you can understand why cholesterol-lowering treatment works so well to prevent heart attacks. When you lower your blood cholesterol level, you don't just stop cholesterol from slowly building up in your arteries; you quickly placate the macrophages that secrete the destructive enzymes responsible for damaging arteries. After a month or two, the cholesterol-filled pockets heal and lose their propensity to burst.

Knowing Your Three Cholesterol Levels

Cholesterol is very sneaky. You can't tell it's getting in your arteries until the damage it does progresses to an advanced stage. That's why it's important not to wait until it causes symptoms. You need to find out if you have high blood cholesterol and correct it before it causes trouble.

You might have heard that your cholesterol level should be less than 200. Forget that. Just knowing your *total* blood cholesterol level is not enough. You need to find out about the three different kinds of cholesterol-containing particles in your blood: bad cholesterol, good cholesterol, and triglyceride.

Bad cholesterol, or low-density lipoprotein (LDL for short), is the stuff that damages your arteries. These particles are just the right size for seeping into artery walls and initiating the chain of events that ultimately leads to damage. Good cholesterol, or high-density lipoprotein (HDL), does the opposite. It cleans out your arteries. These amazing particles act like vacuum cleaners. They suck up cholesterol in your artery walls and carry it back to your liver for disposal. The higher your blood HDL concentration, the better off you are. A one-point increase in your HDL level reduces your risk of heart disease as much as a three-point decrease in your LDL level.

The other cholesterol-containing particle, triglyceride, doesn't get into your artery walls. In fact, in the past, doctors didn't pay much attention to it. The only reason they measured it was to distinguish it from bad cholesterol. However, in recent years triglyceride has gained newfound respect. It turns out that a high triglyceride level is a reliable sign of insulin resistance.

Triglyceride is actually fat traveling from your liver to your fat deposits. If you take in more carbs than your body can handle, your liver turns it to triglyceride and sends it through your bloodstream to your fat deposits for storage. Although triglyceride doesn't damage arteries directly, it depletes HDL, and that depletion does promote cholesterol buildup.

There is, then, a link between diet and heart disease, but it's not through your bad cholesterol levels; it's through your *good* cholesterol. Excessive amounts of refined carbohydrates and lack of exercise aggravate insulin resistance, which raises triglyceride levels, lowers HDL, and increases the risk of heart disease.

How to Tell If You Have a Cholesterol Problem

To tell if you need to take measures to lower your blood cholesterol level, you need to consider not only your bad and good cholesterol levels but also your age, your blood pressure, your family history, and whether you smoke or have diabetes. The National Cholesterol Education Program has developed a simple method for determining whether you have a cholesterol problem.

First, you need to find out your LDL and HDL levels. Your doctor should be able to give you that information over the telephone. Then answer the following questions, and add up your "risk points."

Question	Points
Are you a male 45 years of age or older or a female 55 years of age or older?	Yes = 1; No = 0
Do you smoke cigarettes?	Yes = 1; No = 0
Do you have an immediate family member who has had a heart attack before age 65?	Yes = 1; No = 0
Do you have high blood pressure, or are you being treated for high blood pressure?	Yes = 1; No = 0
Is your HDL level 40 or less if you are a male, or 50 or less if you are a female?	Yes = 1; No = 0
Is your HDL level 60 or greater?	If yes, subtract a point.

Total Points _____

The more of these risk points you have, the lower your LDL level should be to offset the risk. Here's how to tell what your LDL level should be.

- If your score is 0 or 1, your LDL level should be lower than 160.
- If your score is 2 or more, your LDL level should be lower than 130.
- If you have diabetes, your LDL should be lower than 100.
- If you already have artery narrowing or blockage, you should aim for an LDL of 70 or less.

How to Lower Your Blood Cholesterol Level

If you're overweight but your LDL level is safely within the normal range, you can focus your attention on reducing your glycemic load and not worry about cholesterol. However, if according to the National Cholesterol Education Program guidelines your LDL level is higher than it should be, you have two options. You can try to lower it by changing your diet, or you can take cholesterol-lowering medication.

Lowering Cholesterol by Changing Your Diet

If you are overweight and you also have a high LDL level, the first step in changing your diet should be to reduce your intake of refined carbohydrates. "Wait a minute," you might be thinking, "shouldn't I be on a low-cholesterol diet?" Well, to lose weight, you have to cut out starch and sugar anyway, so you might as well see if that lowers your cholesterol. Often it does, especially for people with severe insulin resistance.

However, if eliminating starch and sugar doesn't bring your cholesterol down, you can try going on a low-fat, low-cholesterol diet in addition to cutting out starch and sugar. For most Americans, the main sources of saturated fat and cholesterol are eggs, fatty dairy products such as butter and cheese, and red meat. If you reduce your intake of those foods and eat more unsaturated fat, you might lower your cholesterol levels modestly. (For tips on increasing your intake of "good fats," see Chapter 10.)

Of course, the problem with trying to cut out fat and cholesterol as well as starch and sugar is that it leaves you little else to eat. You might think you have the willpower to do it, but it's hard to cut out bread, potatoes, rice, and sweets in addition to avoiding eggs, meat, and dairy products. Most people can't tolerate the hassle and deprivation of eliminating so many foods for long, and the fact is, it's not a very effective way to lower cholesterol. Low-fat, low-cholesterol diets just don't reduce blood cholesterol levels enough to have much of an effect on most people's risk of heart disease.

Cholesterol-Lowering Medications

If you have high levels of bad cholesterol in your blood, you need to face the fact that you have a genetic quirk. Although most folks would prefer to avoid medications if possible, the reality is that the easiest, most effective way to lower your blood cholesterol level is to take a cholesterol-lowering medication.

You're undoubtedly aware that a lot of people have high blood cholesterol, so you probably wonder if all these folks have genetic quirks. The answer is yes. The human gene pool is riddled with them. Scientists have discovered more than 1,000 different kinds of minor defects in cholesterol metabolism.

Why did Mother Nature allow these quirks to persist? In prehistoric times, it didn't matter what your cholesterol level was. Humans didn't live long enough for cholesterol to accumulate in their arteries. Only since we started living longer has high blood cholesterol affected our longevity.

Medical research has proven that if you have high blood cholesterol, your best bet is to face the fact that you have a genetic quirk in your cholesterol metabolism and take a cholesterol-lowering medication to correct it. One pill a day of a statin type of cholesterol-lowering medication (such as Mevacor, Pravachol, Lescol, Zocor, Lipitor, Crestor, or Vytorin) counteracts the genetic defect that causes high blood cholesterol and allows your body to process it normally. You can then return to eating eggs, meat, and dairy products in moderation and focus your dietary efforts on eliminating starch and sugar—the culprits that most likely caused you to gain weight.

Cholesterol-lowering medications are truly miracle drugs. They have saved more lives than any other drug ever developed. Instead of lowering cholesterol a few percentage points, which is all low-cholesterol diets can usually achieve, statins drop blood cholesterol levels by 40 to 50 percent. Within days, the macrophages in your arteries stop secreting their destructive enzymes, and damaged arteries begin to heal. After a few months, cholesterol buildup recedes, and narrowed arteries often open back up. One cholesterol-lowering pill a day can reduce the risk of heart disease by as much as 67 percent.

The Benefits of a Low-Glycemic-Load Diet

It turns out that a low-glycemic-load diet is a perfect complement to cholesterol-lowering medication. Research shows that when people taking statins switch from a low-cholesterol to a low-glycemic-load diet, even if they eat more fat and cholesterol, their cholesterol balance improves. In one study reported in the journal *Mayo Clinic Proceedings* in 2003, researchers fed subjects who were taking statins a pound and a half of meat and cheese and two to four eggs a day for 6 weeks. Their bad cholesterol levels didn't budge. In fact, the cholesterol particles in their blood became less dense, a quality associated with *reduced* risk of heart disease.

The fact is, if you take a statin, you can go back to eating eggs, meat, and dairy products without worry. This makes it easier to eliminate refined carbohydrates, which relieves insulin resistance, promotes weight loss, and raises HDL—good cholesterol.

The bottom line is this: If you are overweight and you have high blood levels of bad cholesterol, the easiest and most effective way to correct both problems is to focus your dietary and exercise efforts on the carbohydrate side of your metabolism and let medication take care of the cholesterol side.

12

Avoiding Dietary Distractions and Focusing on What's Important

Judy had signs of insulin resistance and was 50 pounds overweight. She understood that she needed to reduce her intake of bread, potatoes, and rice. However, she had been told since childhood that sugar and fat are also bad. She liked eggs, meat, and dairy products but had heard that these are full of cholesterol. In addition, she had read that salt and caffeine could cause high blood pressure. It seemed there was little she *could* eat.

Judy typifies many patients I talk to these days whose efforts to lose weight are hindered by too many dietary distractions. Judy needed to rearrange her priorities to take care of what was most important. The risk to her health posed by large amounts of starch in her diet dwarfed any threat from dietary fat, cholesterol, sugar, salt, or caffeine.

Too Many Distractions

We tend to overestimate our ability to change our diet. Then, when we fall short of our expectations, we get disheartened and quit. The trick to losing weight is to make sure the demands you place on yourself fall within your capabilities. This means focusing on what's throwing your body chemistry out of kilter and on nothing else. There would be little harm in reducing fat, cholesterol, sugar, salt, and caffeine if it didn't interfere with your efforts to lose weight. The problem is that cutting out so many things becomes an unmanageable hassle and leaves too little to enjoy. Face it: If you try to change too much, you will probably tire of the joylessness of the routine and go back to your old ways.

If your blood cholesterol level is okay, there's no point in trying to avoid dietary cholesterol. Even if your cholesterol is high, cutting out cholesterol-containing foods doesn't help much. In fact, it often works against you, because you usually end up eating more carbohydrates. If you really have a cholesterol problem, keeping your level down is truly too important for you to rely on diet. As I discussed in Chapter 11, you're usually better off taking cholesterol-lowering medication.

As for salt and caffeine, avoiding them has not been proven to prevent high blood pressure. Short of medications, the best way to keep your blood pressure down is to keep your weight down. Indeed, the most important lifestyle change you can make for your health in general is to focus on losing weight and avoid being distracted by other dietary concerns.

Focusing on What Caused You to Gain Weight

You've learned that being overweight is not a manifestation of lack of willpower or a self-indulgent personality. It's the result of a hormonal imbalance brought on by the convergence of the following three conditions.

- *A muscle problem:* You have a quirk in your slow-twitch muscle fibers that causes them to fall into a deeper-than-normal dormant state when you don't use them.
- *Long periods of inactivity:* The 20th century lulled you into thinking—as it did most of us—that it's physiologically normal to go for days without walking more than a

few hundred feet at a time. Consequently, your slow-twitch muscle fibers spend too much time turned off to insulin, and your pancreas has to make more insulin than normal to handle the carbohydrates in your diet.

- *Too much starch and sugar:* Economic forces and misdirected fears of fat and cholesterol have driven up the starch and sugar content of your diet to levels your insulin-resistant body can't handle. Repeated glucose shocks make your pancreas secrete huge amounts of insulin, which drives calories into your fat stores and leaves you hungry all the time. In addition, starch short-circuits into your bloodstream in the first foot or two of your intestine and never reaches the last part of your digestive tract, where important appetite-suppressing hormones come from.

So how do you put your body chemistry back in balance? You restore your muscles' sensitivity to insulin by activating your slow-twitch muscle fibers and eliminate glucose shocks by reducing the glycemic load of your diet.

The Lifestyle "Sweet Spot"

Most of us know that exercise promotes weight loss and that starch and sugar are fattening, but often we make the mistake of paying too much attention to one aspect of our metabolism and not enough to another. We might succeed in reducing our glycemic load but fail to activate our slow-twitch muscle fibers. Or we might exercise regularly but continue to assail our bodies with glucose shocks.

You can lose weight by lowering your glycemic load or by exercising, but the easiest way is to do both. Athletes talk about being "in the zone" or finding the "sweet spot" where they perform their best. Similarly, if you just eliminate the major dietary offenders and do just enough of the right kind of exercise, your metabolism will enter a "zone" where it performs best. Your insulin levels will drop like a rock, and without your going hungry or engaging in grueling exercise, your body chemistry will start humming again. Fat should melt away effortlessly.

Taking Inventory

To know where best to apply your effort, it might help to take inventory of the state of your body chemistry. This section will help you answer the following questions.

- How much is your weight affecting your health?
- How insulin resistant are you?
- How much time do your slow-twitch muscle fibers spend in the sleep mode?
- What is the glycemic load of your diet?
- Do you have high blood cholesterol?

Knowing what aspects of your body chemistry are abnormal will help you put your metabolism back in balance with as little effort and disruption of your life as possible.

How Much Is Your Weight Affecting Your Health?

From the standpoint of appearance, the definition of overweight depends on personal preference and the fashion of the day. However, for the sake of your health, you need to know how much your weight is affecting your metabolism. Excess body fat triggers a vicious cycle: It worsens insulin resistance, and insulin resistance, in turn, promotes more weight gain. The more overweight you are, the worse your insulin resistance, and the more you need to focus on relieving it.

A good way to judge how much your weight is affecting your metabolism is to look at statistics relating body weight to diseases caused by insulin resistance, such as diabetes and heart disease. Scientists have devised a formula for judging risk using height and weight measurements. They call it the *body mass index* (BMI). To estimate your risk, first find your BMI in Table 12.1 by looking at your height and weight.

Regardless of your gender, most doctors regard a BMI of 24 or lower as being ideal, 25 to 29 as mildly overweight, 30 to 34 as markedly overweight, and 35 or higher as obese. Once you know your BMI, you can use Figure 12.1 (opposite) to determine your risk of obesity-related diseases.

Table 12.1 Body Mass Index Table

	Normal		Moderately Overweight					Markedly Overweight						Obese				
BMI	**23**	**24**	**25**	**26**	**27**	**28**	**29**	**30**	**31**	**32**	**33**	**34**	**35**	**36**	**37**	**38**	**39**	**40**
								Body Weight (pounds)										
58	110	115	119	124	129	134	138	143	148	153	158	162	167	172	177	181	186	191
59	114	119	124	128	133	138	143	148	153	158	163	168	173	178	183	188	193	198
60	118	123	128	133	138	143	148	153	158	163	168	174	179	184	189	194	199	204
61	122	127	132	137	143	148	153	158	164	169	174	180	185	190	195	201	206	211
62	126	131	136	142	147	153	158	164	169	175	180	186	191	196	202	207	213	218
63	130	135	141	146	152	158	163	169	175	180	186	191	197	203	208	214	220	225
64	134	140	145	151	157	163	169	174	180	186	192	197	204	209	215	221	227	232
65	138	144	150	156	162	168	174	180	186	192	198	204	210	216	222	228	234	240
66	142	148	155	161	167	173	179	186	192	198	204	210	216	223	229	235	241	247
67	146	153	159	166	172	178	185	191	198	204	211	217	223	230	236	242	249	255
68	151	158	164	171	177	184	190	197	203	210	216	223	230	236	243	249	256	262
69	155	162	169	176	182	189	196	203	209	216	223	230	236	243	250	257	263	270
70	160	167	174	181	188	195	202	209	216	222	229	236	243	250	257	264	271	278
71	165	172	179	186	193	200	208	215	222	229	236	243	250	257	265	272	279	286
72	169	177	184	191	199	206	213	221	228	235	242	250	258	265	272	279	287	294
73	174	182	189	197	204	212	219	227	235	242	250	257	265	272	280	288	295	302
74	179	186	194	202	210	218	225	233	241	249	256	264	272	280	287	295	303	311
75	184	192	200	208	216	224	232	240	248	256	264	272	279	287	295	303	311	319
76	189	197	205	213	221	230	238	246	254	263	271	279	287	295	304	312	320	328

Height (inches) is listed vertically along the left side.

Source: National Heart, Lung, and Blood Institute (nhlbi.nih.gov/guidelines/obesity)

Figure 12.1 Cardiovascular Risk According to Body Mass Index

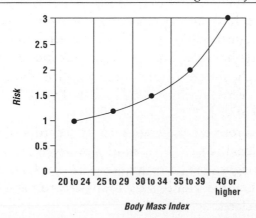

As you can see, the more you weigh, the higher your risk of diabetes and heart disease. Notice that if your BMI is lower than 25, the effect of a few extra pounds is negligible. The risk starts rising above 25, and beyond 30, your chance of developing diabetes or heart disease skyrockets.

How Insulin Resistant Are You?

Some overweight individuals have worse insulin resistance than others do. An amazingly simple yet accurate way to tell how insulin resistant you are is to measure your abdominal circumference at the level of your navel. (*Note:* Use a tape measure. Do not rely on pants size.)

- Regardless of your height, if your girth measured at your navel is more than 38 inches if you're a male or 34 inches if you're a female, your risk of diabetes doubles.
- If your girth is more than 40 inches if you're a male or 36 inches if you're a female, your risk of diabetes triples.
- If your girth is more than 42 inches if you're a male or 38 inches if you're a female, your risk of diabetes quadruples.

The good news is that the worse your insulin resistance, the more dramatically it will improve when you correct the factors that cause it. If you concentrate on reducing your glycemic load and activating your slow-twitch muscle fibers, your body shape will quickly change. Your abdomen will shrink before the rest of you does. In fact, the best way to monitor your progress in reversing insulin resistance is not to follow your weight, since you might gain muscle as you lose fat. Just notice the way your pants fit.

How Much Time Do Your Slow-Twitch Muscle Fibers Spend in the Sleep Mode?

As I discussed in Chapter 8, it takes 20 to 30 minutes of steady aerobic activity like walking or jogging to get your slow-twitch muscles to wake up and start responding to insulin. After a few hours, they slowly begin losing sensitivity, and in 48 hours, they're back where they started. Thus, the more often you go longer than 48 hours without exercise, the more time your body spends in an insulin-resistant state.

More than 1 or 2 days a week of insulin resistance will raise your risk of obesity and diabetes. This means that in order to eliminate insulin resistance periods, you need to exercise at least every other day—that's four times a week at regular intervals. Research studies consistently show that this is the frequency of exercise needed to lose weight and prevent diabetes. However, if you have a low fidget factor (for example, if you spend more than 6 hours a day in front of a computer or a television screen), you should probably exercise as many days in a week as you spend engaged in sedentary activities.

What Is the Glycemic Load of Your Diet?

You can gauge how much insulin your body has to make by adding up the glycemic loads of the foods you eat. According to research linking diet with diabetes and heart disease, most people can handle a glycemic load of up to approximately 500 a day without harmful insulin excess. However, a daily tally greater than 500 will drive up your insulin levels and promote weight gain.

As I mentioned in Chapter 4, you shouldn't need a list of glycemic load ratings of foods to tell whether your glycemic load is too high. There are only a few culprits: bread, potatoes, rice, breakfast cereal, pasta, and sugar-containing soft drinks. You can probably get away with eating one average-size serving of one of these offenders a day, but more than that, when added to the smaller glycemic loads you get in other foods, is usually enough to push your glycemic load above 500. More than two full servings a day of starch will definitely promote weight gain and increase your risk of diabetes and heart disease.

Do You Have High Blood Cholesterol?

High blood cholesterol is a silent killer. It causes no symptoms until it reaches an advanced stage. You can be thin and physically fit but still have a dangerously high cholesterol level. As you learned in Chapter 11, the only way to tell if you have a cholesterol problem is to measure the levels of the three different kinds of cholesterol particles in your blood. If, according to the National Cholesterol Education Program guidelines, your bad cholesterol level is too high, you probably have a genetic quirk in your body's mechanisms for removing cholesterol. This can only mean trouble. In addition to losing weight, you need to find a fail-safe means of keeping your blood cholesterol level down.

You've learned that the way your body handles carbohydrates and its ability to remove cholesterol from your blood are two separate aspects of your metabolism. How your body metabolizes carbs depends largely on your diet and physical activity patterns. Your cholesterol level depends on how efficient your system is at removing cholesterol, and your genes determine this. The easiest and most effective way to put your body chemistry back in balance is to use medications if necessary to lower cholesterol, and devote your dietary and exercise efforts toward relieving insulin resistance.

The Rewards

If you do what you need to do to alleviate insulin resistance—eliminate glucose shocks and activate your slow-twitch muscle fibers—even if you don't try to cut calories, remarkable things will happen.

- *You will usually lose weight without dieting.* Eliminating the dietary culprits that cause your body to overproduce insulin removes little in the way of richness and flavor from your diet. You can eat satisfying amounts of good food and still lose weight.
- *You will reduce your risk of diabetes.* When you reduce the amount of insulin your pancreas has to make, you reduce your risk of type 2 diabetes.
- *If you already have type 2 diabetes, it will improve dramatically.* If you combine standard medication for type 2 diabetes with the program described in this book, chances are your blood glucose levels will return to normal. (*Caution:* If you are already taking medication for diabetes, the dosages needed might decline significantly, causing

your blood glucose levels to fall too low. You should monitor your blood glucose closely and discuss your treatment
with your doctor.)

- *Your cholesterol profile will improve.* Although relieving
insulin resistance usually doesn't reduce bad cholesterol
levels much, it dramatically lowers blood triglyceride levels
and raises the concentrations of protective cholesterol,
HDL, in your blood. This improves the balance between
good and bad cholesterol and reduces your risk of heart and
blood vessel disease.

- *Your mood will improve.* Improving the way your body
handles carbohydrates will soften the adrenaline fluctuations that jerk your nerves back and forth from being jan-
gled to burned out. Your mood, concentration, and energy
levels will improve noticeably.

Freedom from Dieting

Crash dieters often experience a sense of impending disappoint-
ment, as if they expect their house of cards to come tumbling
down at any time, which, in fact, it usually does. It's a different
story for people who understand insulin resistance and do what
they need to do to relieve it. They exude the confidence of someone
who "gets it." They have a clear vision of what they are trying to
accomplish, and they know the difference between what they can
change and what they cannot.

Losing weight by reducing the glycemic load of your diet and
targeting your physical activity toward sensitizing your muscles to
insulin bears little resemblance to the timeworn approach of starving yourself and sweating off pounds. As you will see in the next
chapter of this book—where you'll find great ideas for meals and
delicious recipes—you can eat heartily, feel satisfied, and reduce
your glycemic load.

13

Grocery Shopping and Eating Out

Several years ago, I discovered I had a reason to reduce my own glycemic load. I had type 1 diabetes. My initial reaction was one of dismay. I thought my fine-dining days were over. I soon came to realize I was wrong.

Back when we were told we should cut down on fat and cholesterol, I followed the party line and tried to avoid eggs, red meat, and dairy products. However, by the time I developed diabetes, it was becoming apparent that these foods were not as bad as everyone thought. They really weren't what caused high blood cholesterol, and unlike carbohydrates, they didn't raise blood sugar. I discovered I could enjoy them in abundance, and my blood cholesterol levels were lower than ever. All I had to do was concentrate on carbohydrates.

A More Exciting Way to Eat

Initially, cutting out carbs looked like a big job, but once I became familiar with the concept of glycemic load, I realized there were only a handful of carbohydrates I needed to cut out: grain products, potatoes, rice, and soft drinks. I could even enjoy sweets in moderation, as long as they weren't starchy ones.

I also discovered there's a bonus to reducing your glycemic load: When you stop eating bread, potatoes, and rice with every meal, you make room for more variety and flavor. Truthfully, I eat heartier now than I did before.

Of course, if someone tells you that you shouldn't eat something, you start thinking you can't live without it. But honestly, is starch so wonderful you're willing to sacrifice your health and your looks for it? Bread, potatoes, and rice are "comfort foods." Because they were among the first foods our mothers fed us, they presumably evoke feelings of warmth and security. But humans have no biological need for starch and no natural craving for it. Getting the tasteless paste out of your diet makes room for healthier food and more exciting tastes and textures.

So forget about depriving yourself. Consider this an opportunity to broaden your palate and embark upon a culinary adventure. Here are some suggestions to help you get started.

- *Don't throw away your old cookbooks.* The day after I told my wife I had diabetes, she made a trip to the bookstore to buy diabetic cookbooks. Later, we realized there's no need to invest in special cookbooks to follow a low-glycemic-load diet. Virtually all of the cookbooks she already had offered a wealth of starch-free dishes. If you don't own a cookbook, forget about diet cookbooks. Make your first purchase a classic like the *Joy of Cooking* or *The Silver Palate Cookbook.*
- *Learn how to recognize starch in recipes.* Spotting starch is simple. It's always visible and rarely blended with other ingredients. Look for recipes that contain no crusts, breading, potatoes, or rice. A tablespoon or two of flour or a half cup of bread crumbs to hold other ingredients together won't hurt. Neither should a few teaspoons of sugar in an otherwise starch-free dish. Just avoid large hunks of starch.
- *Remember that "low carb" is not the same as "low glycemic load."* Most of the recipes in low-carb cookbooks are fine. However, many of these books go too far in eliminating

fruits, vegetables, milk products, and sugar but not far enough in getting rid of starch. Some purportedly low-carb recipes contain significant amounts of ingredients you should avoid, such as whole grain flour and brown rice. Although these less refined starches contain more vitamins and fiber than their whiter versions do, they're just as bad when it comes to causing glucose shocks.

To assemble a repertoire of great low-glycemic-load recipes, I enlisted the help of two nationally recognized nutrition experts and cookbook authors.

Dana Carpender has published several best-selling cookbooks, including *500 Low-Carb Recipes* and *Dana Carpender's Every Calorie Counts Cookbook*. For years, she had a nationwide syndicated newspaper column. I have been impressed with Dana's extensive knowledge of food preparation and her fine food sense. Dana understands how new knowledge about nutrition can set food lovers free.

Molly Siple, nutrition editor of *Natural Health* magazine, a registered dietitian, and author of several popular cookbooks, provided a couple of dozen of her favorite recipes, which capture the spirit of the low-glycemic-load style of eating.

Before we get to the recipes, though, here is a variety of information that will make shifting over to a low-glycemic-load lifestyle easier for you. You can also turn to Appendix A on page 330 to see the glycemic loads of more than 150 foods, and then Appendix B on page 340 for a 2-week meal plan that will keep your glycemic load under 500 a day, which is your overall goal.

Convenience Foods

Chances are you're not a "foodie." Up until you realized your health depended on changing your eating habits, you probably depended on the same packaged, processed convenience foods that everyone else eats. You know, don't you, that you can't rely on all this starchy garbage anymore?

"But," you protest, "I have a job! I have kids! I have a million things to do! I don't always have time to cook!" Or maybe you simply hate to cook and have picked up this book out of desperation over your health issues.

Good news: There are convenience foods that fit the glycemic load diet. Your menu will be more interesting if you cook, but you don't *have* to.

These convenience foods may put a ding in your budget. Unlike the convenience foods you're used to, these aren't based on cheap starch. But you know what? Food that makes you fat, sick, tired, and hungry wouldn't be cheap if they were giving it away.

Here are some great convenience foods that work for the glycemic load diet.

In the Deli

- **Rotisserie chicken.** The ultimate low-glycemic-load convenience food. A rotisserie chicken plus bagged salad makes a quick and satisfying supper.
- **Deli meats.** Great for low-carb tortilla wraps, of course, but also try unsandwiches—spread your condiments between a couple of slices of cold cuts and roll them up inside a lettuce leaf, along with a slice of tomato, if you like.
- **Deli salads and vegetables.** Skip the potato and macaroni salads. Look for coleslaw, roasted vegetables, sautéed green beans in olive oil, and other interesting vegetable dishes. And don't forget chicken salad and tuna salad.

In the Freezer Case

- **Frozen hot wings.** Nuke and eat. Watch out for breading.
- **Frozen hamburger patties.** Read the label to avoid starchy fillers.
- **Frozen grilled fish fillets.** These come with garlic butter, Cajun seasoning, lemon pepper, Italian herbs, and other seasonings.
- **Frozen vegetables.** I know fresh vegetables are the choice of gourmets everywhere, but I'm in favor of anything that gets you and your family to eat your darned vegetables. Just microwave, butter, and eat. Great for soups and stews too.

And with a bag of stir-fry blend and some boneless, skinless chicken in the freezer, plus a bottle of your favorite stir-fry sauce on the shelf, you're never more than 10 minutes away from a great meal. Be careful, though. More and more frozen vegetable blends include noodles and other starchy ingredients. Be clear on what you're getting.

- **Frozen fruit.** Frozen fruit of every kind is great to keep on hand for smoothies or for tossing into yogurt. In the winter, the frozen ones are often better than the fresh ones anyway. Use frozen unsweetened peach slices in any recipe that calls for cooking the peaches. It's a lot easier than peeling and slicing all those peaches!

In the Meat and Fish Department

- **Preskewered kebabs.** Just throw them on the grill or under the broiler.
- **Precooked ham and turkey ham.** The kind in a big oval chunk. Brown a slice or two in butter to eat with eggs or cut cubes to scramble into them. Brown a slice of ham per customer in butter, flip, and while the other side is browning, spread the top with mustard and cover with Swiss or Cheddar cheese. Or just cut off a slice and stuff it in your face.
- **Cooked chicken breast strips.** Great for tossing in a salad, filling an omelet, or making a wrap in a low-carb tortilla.
- **Precooked shrimp.** Toss into a salad or dip in cocktail sauce.
- **Precooked crab legs.** Dip in cocktail sauce or go for the lemon butter.
- **Precooked bacon.** I haven't tried this, but I know people who swear by it. The best part, they say, is that you don't have all that grease to deal with.

In the Canned Meat Aisle

- **Canned or pouch-pack tuna.** Tuna salad takes 5 minutes to throw together. Bagged salad tossed with bottled dressing and topped with tuna is even quicker. Tuna now comes in various flavors, by the way, but read the labels and watch out for starchy additives.

- **Canned crab, chicken, chunk ham, and salmon.** See the tuna suggestions above.
- **Smoked salmon.** Put it in an omelet or serve it on a salad.

In the Dairy Case

- **Eggs.** It's hard to think of a way to cook eggs that takes more than 20 minutes. In particular, if you like hard-cooked eggs, keep some in the fridge at all times, ready to grab.
- **Individually wrapped cheese sticks and chunks.** These make a terrific grab-and-go breakfast or emergency rations in your purse or attaché case, though you wouldn't want to keep them in there longer than a day, of course.
- **Cottage cheese in single-serving containers with peel-off lids.** Throw one in your purse with a plastic spoon and there's breakfast. Or lunch, for that matter.
- **Sugar-free yogurt in tons of flavors.** Sugary yogurt is too close to sugared beverages to be a good idea. But artificially sweetened yogurt now comes in a wide variety of flavors, and it couldn't be easier to grab and eat.

In the Produce Department

- **Precut carrots, celery, broccoli, and cauliflower.** You know, all the stuff you find on a relish tray. A plate of these plus some ranch dip makes a salad or cooked vegetable unnecessary. It's a great idea to set this out as soon as you get home, for the whole family to snack on. Beats letting them fill up on chips. Grab some **grape or cherry tomatoes** while you're at it.
- **Bagged salad.** The greatest development in packaged foods in the last 50 years. Buy it. Eat it. And don't forget to try a new blend now and then.
- **Precut fruit.** Chunks of melon and pineapple, even mango. Good for snacking or fruit salad. Stash 'em in the freezer for a chilly summer treat or to throw into smoothies.
- **Salad bar items.** You can make salad at the grocery store salad bar, of course. But it's also a great source of pre-prepped vegetables for stir-fries and other uses.

- **Guacamole.** You may be walking past the guacamole because you don't know how to eat it without chips. Stuff it into a tomato for a killer salad! Use it to top a steak or grilled chicken breast. Combine it with Monterey Jack for the world's yummiest omelet filling.
- **Prechopped onions.** Many grocery stores carry chopped fresh onions in plastic tubs. These can streamline everything from chili to stir-fries to slow-cooker meals.
- **Presliced mushrooms.** Sliced fresh mushrooms cost the same as unsliced. Why do the work?
- **Prechopped "stoplight" peppers.** Mixed chopped yellow, red, and green peppers in plastic tubs. Throw 'em in a salad, use 'em in a stir-fry—whatever you might want chopped peppers for.

Eating Out

Keeping your glycemic load low while eating out is easy. We've shunned bread, rice, potatoes, and pasta for 13 years now, and we have rarely found a restaurant where I couldn't order a meal that fit my dietary needs and tasted great too.

Four notes, the first of which is the most important:

- **Ask for what you want.** Restaurants are in a service industry; reasonable requests should be met cheerfully. It's a rare restaurant that won't substitute an extra serving of vegetables or side salad for the rice or potato. If a restaurant will not accommodate reasonable special orders, take your business elsewhere.
- **Ask questions!** If you're not sure whether a dish is appropriate, ask what's in it. Is it breaded? Is it battered? Is the soup thickened with flour or cornstarch? A good waiter will know or offer to find out. Fast-food restaurants usually have a chart of ingredients and nutritional values somewhere; ask.
- **Have the waiter take the bread basket away unless the other diners object.** Why tempt yourself, especially when you're hungry? Save your appetite for the good stuff.

- **If the starch offered with your meal is very special,** a real personal favorite of yours, here's what we suggest: Have the waiter bring it, but leave it by the side of your plate. Eat the rest of your meal—the protein, the vegetables, the salad—all that great stuff. If you're still hungry for the starchy food at the end of your meal, eat about a quarter of it. This works, of course, only if you've got what it takes to have a few bites and leave the rest. If you know that one bite will lead to devouring the whole thing, better to ask the waiter to leave it off your plate altogether.

Standard American

Your Applebee's/Ruby Tuesday/T.G.I. Friday's sort of place. They're a cinch. Get a steak, ribs, grilled chops. Watch out for breaded "crispy" chicken, but if they have grilled or roasted chicken, that's great too. These places also have a good selection of main-dish salads, which are perfect for us. Read carefully to determine whether the chicken in salads is grilled or crispy—i.e., breaded and fried. Even if the menu specifies crispy chicken, restaurants should substitute grilled chicken on request.

Barbecue Joint

Hey, it's slow-smoked meat. That's for you! Ribs, chicken, beef brisket, you name it, you can eat it. If your 'cue is seasoned with dry rub, it's perfect. If it has sauce (mmmm—barbecue sauce . . .), go easy; most barbecue sauce is very sugary. Feel free to eat the slaw and greens, but skip the fries, hush puppies, cornbread, and baked beans. Have another rib instead. Are you a pulled pork fan? Instead of having a sandwich, pile your pulled pork on top of a big plate of slaw, an incredible combination.

Chinese

Easy! Start with spareribs, egg drop soup, or hot and sour soup instead of an egg roll, wonton, or shrimp toast. Most stir-fries are perfect for us, since they consist of meat and vegetables. Skip the rice. Be wary of sweet-and-sour dishes; the meat is usually battered. Skip the moo shu pancakes too. (If you're taking your Chinese food home, you can use low-carb tortillas in place of the moo shu pancakes. They work nicely.)

Corner Coffee Shops and Diners

You know the kind of place—with the rotating case of desserts up front and the waitresses who call you "hon." These places have good salads, starting with the old classic chef's salad. Often they have a "diet plate" consisting of a bunless hamburger patty and a scoop of cottage cheese, which has been on the menu since back before low-fat mania hit, when everyone knew that if you wanted to lose weight, you ate protein, not starch.

Often you can get a steak, grilled pork chops, half a grilled chicken, and other good entrées. Ask for an extra salad or veggies in place of the potato. They'll probably have good slaw too. Many coffee shops and diners serve breakfast 'round the clock, and they often have an impressive selection of egg dishes. Nothing like a big omelet or steak and eggs (hold the toast and the hash browns) to fill you up.

Deli

The traditional Jewish or Italian deli can be a 50-50 proposition: You can have any kind of cold cuts they sell; you just can't have them on bread or a roll. Fortunately, most delis offer salads too. Ask for all the innards of your favorite sandwich served on a bed of lettuce. Delis also offer great tuna or chicken salad—eat it with a fork, not as a sandwich. You will, of course, ignore the potato and macaroni salads.

Instead of getting a bread basket while you wait for your meal (and admittedly, Jewish breads and rolls are wonderful), you can almost always get a dish of kosher pickles to nosh on.

Greek

Try ordering all the insides of a gyros sandwich served on top of a Greek salad instead of in a pita. Terrific! Stuffed grape leaves are popular but usually have rice in the filling; sample just one if you must. Skip the starchy hummus; have tzatziki (cucumber-yogurt dip) instead. Dip veggies in it, not pita. Feel free to devour feta and olives.

Moussaka is likely to have bread crumbs in the meat mixture and is topped with a starch-thickened sauce, so skip it. Stick to the roasted or grilled meat and poultry dishes. Greek roasted chicken is legendary, as are Greek lamb kebabs and pork souvlaki. There are likely to be excellent vegetable dishes available as well—Greek green beans, cooked in tomato sauce, are especially good.

Italian

Italian restaurants can be rough. This is changing, though; many now offer grilled chicken and fish dishes. Do the best you can. If they offer the traditional chicken cacciatore—chicken stewed in tomato sauce with peppers, onions, and mushrooms—it's a fine choice.

Every Italian meal comes with at least a side of pasta, but that's easy to fix; ask for salad or steamed veggies instead. If they offer all-you-can-eat salad, hey, eat all you can! But skip the all-you-can-eat breadsticks and the garlic bread. Skip the soup as well; most Italian soups contain starchy beans or pasta or both.

Many Italian restaurants now offer excellent main-dish salads. Hot cheese dips—spinach-artichoke-mozzarella dip and the like—are currently trendy on Italian menus. With raw vegetables instead of bread for dipping, this can make a satisfying light meal.

Japanese

Sashimi is perfect; sushi has too much rice. Miso soup is fine. Teppanyaki-style grilled meat, poultry, fish, and/or vegetable dishes are ideal. Stir-fries are fine too. Skip rice, noodles, and dumplings. Avoid tempura, because of the batter.

Mexican

Like Italian restaurants, Mexican restaurants lean toward big doses of starch, starting with that basket of chips. As with the bread basket, it's best simply to ask the waiter to take the chips away.

Mexican restaurants often have good main-dish salads, but watch out for tortilla strips, beans, and corn. Fajitas are perfect; just eat them with a fork instead of in a tortilla. Grilled beef dishes like puntas de filete and carne asada are easy to find, as are grilled shrimp and chicken dishes. Mexican stews are good and usually don't contain potatoes. Carnitas—meltingly tender chunks of simmered and then browned pork—are fantastic.

Speaking of guacamole, it's not only delicious but great for you. Order extra and pile it on salads, fajitas, steaks—or just eat it with a fork. You should steer clear of tortillas, rice, and refried beans. This rules out tacos, burritos, enchiladas, chimichangas, and flautas. Sorry!

Pizza Parlor

Thick-crust pan pizza is out! You can get the thinnest-crust pizza you can find and leave the thick edge behind. Or you can order your pizza with a ton of toppings—extra cheese, pepperoni, sausage, peppers, mushrooms, anchovies, whatever you want. Then peel those toppings off the crust and scarf them down, leaving the starchy crust behind. (It helps if the pizza's had a couple of minutes to cool. Then the cheese pulls off in a solid layer, with all the other stuff attached.) The toppings are the good part, anyway. The crust is just an edible napkin.

Many pizza places have good salads, with Italian vinaigrette dressing and lots of red onion and olives, and those pickled hot peppers. There's your side dish, if you want one.

You know that stuff like "cheesy bread," breadsticks, garlic bread, etc., is out. Pizza places love to load you up on this stuff to make it look like you're getting a great value, but that white flour cost them next to nothing—and will cost you big-time.

Seafood

If you're a seafood fan, this is one of the best possible types of restaurants for you. Any grilled, steamed, boiled, baked, or sautéed fish or seafood is likely to be fine. Just watch out for dishes that are breaded and fried, baked dishes topped with bread crumbs, and any dish in which the fish is combined with pasta or rice. You'll skip the baked potato and the bread basket, of course. But feel free to dip your lobster and crab in melted butter!

Steak House

Can it get any better than a steak house for a low-glycemic-load diet? Any steak you want is just fine. These places often have chicken and seafood too, but again, watch out for breading. Of course you'll skip the baked potato or fries. Ask for an extra salad or order of steamed veggies instead. And those "onion blossom" things or the more common onion rings? They're crack in food form, but they're also coated in batter. If you can't limit yourself to one or two, better to avoid them altogether.

Steak houses often have salad bars. All the vegetables are fine, of course. So is any fresh fruit they may offer. Skip the croutons and Chinese noodles—if you want a little crunch, sunflower seeds or bacon bits are better choices. Pretend the pasta, potato, and bean salads aren't there.

Fast Food

Contrary to popular belief, it is possible to eat fast food and be perfectly healthy. Most fast-food places offer low-glycemic-load options—it's up to you to choose them! However, if the smell of fryer grease goes to your head and you can't get out of a fast-food joint without eating fries or gulping a shake, you'd do better to simply stay away.

Here's a quick rundown of the low-glycemic-load options at the most popular fast-food places.

McDonald's, Burger King, Wendy's, Jack in the Box, and Arby's all offer main-dish salads. These are the obvious choice. Often you'll have the choice of grilled or crispy chicken—remember that *crispy* means "breaded"—so go for the grilled chicken. Leave off starchy toppers like croutons and Chinese noodles. You can, of course, also have a burger without the bun on top of a side salad.

Hardee's has no salads, but its West Coast version, Carl's Jr., offers a charbroiled chicken salad, perfect for us. Both Hardee's and Carl's Jr. offer particularly big hamburger patties, nice when you're leaving off the bun. You might ask for extra lettuce and tomatoes. Carl's Jr. also has a burger with sautéed portobello mushrooms, which sounds darn good to me! Hardee's and Carl's Jr. both offer chargrilled chicken sandwiches. Again, leave off the bun, ask for extra lettuce, tomatoes, and mayo, and you've got a simple but healthful meal.

If you're lucky enough to live in In-N-Out Burger territory, you can order its famous burgers "protein style"—wrapped in lettuce.

White Castle is a dead loss, not a thing for us on the menu. I've never been able to fathom the popularity of "sliders" anyway—those hamburger patties are the size of postage stamps. Go somewhere where they're more generous with the protein.

Taco Bell has only one low-glycemic-load selection: Order a taco salad, either beef or chicken. Ask them to hold the beans and double the meat. Then don't eat the taco shell! (If you can't resist the taco shell, best go elsewhere.)

Subway is a great choice. All of its sandwich fillings can be ordered as salads, with lettuce, cucumbers, peppers, and other great veggies added. Quizno's is Subway's biggest competitor. It offers five main-dish salads. Just ignore the little triangles of flatbread stuck in the sides—or if your will is weak, ask them to hold the bread. Quizno's also has a broccoli-cheese soup that should be reasonably okay for us.

Long John Silver's manages to make fish unhealthful; most its selections are breaded and fried, and with the exception of coleslaw, all the side dishes are starchy. Go somewhere else.

KFC has a couple of main-dish salads on the menu, available with either roasted or crispy chicken. Choose the roasted chicken. There are also a few side dishes at KFC that are okay—the slaw, the green beans, and the side salad.

Popeyes also offers only breaded and fried chicken. Its seafood is breaded and fried as well. Some Popeyes offer a shrimp Creole that should be okay if you get it without the rice, but that's about it—they don't even have main-dish salads.

If you live in Boston Market territory, it's one of your best choices. You can get roasted chicken or turkey and even roast sirloin. Boston Market has salads and slaw, green beans, steamed mixed vegetables tossed in olive oil, spinach in garlic butter, and creamed spinach.

Kenny Rogers Roasters, similar to Boston Market, offers plenty of good choices—roasted chicken, of course, but also roasted turkey and barbecued ribs. (Go easy on the sugary barbecue sauce.) They have main-dish and side salads, herbed Italian green beans, creamy spinach with Parmesan, grilled vegetables, and mixed peas and carrots too.

Chick-fil-A offers a couple of chargrilled chicken salads that are fine. It also has fruit salad, coleslaw, "chicken salad cups," and side salads. Avoid the "chicken strips" salad; the chicken is breaded and fried.

Low-Glycemic-Load Cooking: Easy and Delicious

Try some of the recipes on the following pages, or even just read about them, and you'll see that reducing your glycemic load can be the key to a richer, more enjoyable way of eating.

Of course, all you have to do is look around you to find good low-glycemic-load recipes. Kathy Casey, author of *Pacific Northwest: The Beautiful Cookbook* and *Dishing with Kathy Casey,* contributed a few of her favorite low-glycemic-load recipes. My wife, a great cook, also added a few of our favorite dishes. You will find, however, that there's really no need for special food preparation to follow a low-glycemic-load eating style. In each food category, I have listed several classic dishes you can easily find in most cookbooks and frequently on restaurant menus.

A Few Ingredients You Should Know About

Shirataki Noodles: There is one truly low-starch noodle. Indeed, it's a low-*everything* noodle. Let me introduce you to shirataki. Shirataki noodles are made of virtually nothing but fiber and water. The shirataki in my fridge claim to have 1 gram of carbohydrate, 1 gram of fiber, and no calories at all.

There are two varieties of shirataki noodles, traditional and tofu shirataki. The traditional noodles are clear, with a jellylike consistency and very little flavor of their own. They are distinctively Asian. As a result, they really work only in Asian dishes—they were truly weird with tomato sauce and Parmesan. But they're a great choice for sesame noodles, pad Thai, Asian noodles and broth, you name it.

Tofu shirataki are white and have a consistency that is closer to that of wheat noodles. They too are quite bland. They're the noodles to choose if you're making more traditional Western-style dishes. I've made fettuccine Alfredo and a very good mac and cheese with the tofu shirataki. They're also good in tuna-noodle casserole. Tofu shirataki come in two widths, spaghetti width and fettuccine width.

Both traditional and tofu shirataki come already hydrated, in a plastic pouch full of liquid. To use them, you snip the pouch open and pour the noodles into a strainer in your sink to drain. You will notice that the liquid smells fishy. Panic not. Soaking the noodles in warm water for 20 minutes or so—while you assemble the rest of your dish—will dispel the smell. I haven't noticed the noodles actually tasting fishy.

Shirataki noodles are a lot longer than the spaghetti and fettuccine you're used to, and the traditional version resists being bitten off! So take your kitchen shears and snip, willy-nilly, across the mass of noodles four or five times. This will take care of the problem.

Find shirataki noodles at Asian markets and some health food stores. Shirataki can be ordered from Internet retailers as well. They keep for up to a year if refrigerated, so feel free to stock up.

Guar or Xanthan: You've been eating guar and xanthan all your life. They're widely used in the food-processing industry, as thickeners—which is exactly how you're going to use them.

Sauces, gravies, soups, stir-fries, and many other dishes call for flour, cornstarch, or arrowroot as thickeners. But all of those are starches, and highly refined starches at that. Guar and xanthan are instead finely milled, tasteless soluble fibers. They give a nice, velvety texture to gravies, soups, and sauces and add no flavor of their own.

Guar and xanthan are very similar; use them interchangeably. The easiest way to use whichever you buy is to keep it in an old saltshaker by the stove. When your sauce, soup, or gravy needs thickening, simply sprinkle the guar or xanthan lightly over the top, whisking as you do so. Stop when your dish is just a little less thick than you'd like it to be, since it will continue to thicken a little on standing.

What you should *not* do is dump a spoonful of guar or xanthan into your dish, then try to whisk it in. You'll get a big lump of jellylike stuff in the middle of your food.

Guar and xanthan are available at health food stores and online. A little goes a long way, so you shouldn't have to repurchase often. And they keep forever, as long as they don't get wet.

Vital Wheat Gluten: Gluten is a protein found in grains. When you add moisture and knead gluten, it becomes stretchy. It's that stretchy quality that allows bread dough to hold in the carbon dioxide created by growing yeast in a billion tiny bubbles, making bread rise. Rye, oats, and barley have a little gluten in them, but wheat has the most. This is why most recipes, even for rye or oatmeal bread, call for at least some wheat flour too.

But you can't use more than a little bit of wheat flour because of all that starch. The good news is you can replace much of it with fiber and protein powder. So use separated gluten, or *vital wheat gluten*, to replace the starchy regular flour.

The labeling on vital wheat gluten can be confusing. Some companies label it *vital wheat gluten,* while others just call it *wheat gluten* or *gluten*. Others call it *gluten flour,* but usually gluten flour is starchy white flour with some extra gluten added to it. How to tell? Read the label. A quarter cup of vital wheat gluten should have about 47 grams of protein and only about 3 grams of carbohydrate.

Gluten sensitivity is common; it's one of the reasons grains are not great foods for many people. Find vital wheat gluten at health food stores and sometimes in the baking aisle of big grocery stores. I use Bob's Red Mill brand.

Vanilla Whey Protein: Whey is the liquid part of milk. Protein powder made from whey is extremely nutritious, has a mild flavor, and works well for making smoothies and for replacing part of the flour in a lot of recipes. You can buy vanilla whey protein at health food stores, GNC stores, and anywhere that sells supplements for bodybuilders.

Rice Protein Powder: Rice protein powder is useful in savory dishes, where vanilla whey would taste funny. We use NutriBiotic brand, which we special-order through our health food store. If your health food store doesn't have rice protein powder, no doubt it can special-order it for you too.

Almond Meal: Almond meal is useful as a substitute for flour and cornmeal. Many grocery stores carry almond meal; check the baking aisle. However, almond meal is simple to make yourself. Just dump shelled almonds into your food processor and run it till you have a meal about the texture of coarse cornmeal.

Store almond meal in an airtight container or resealable plastic bag in the fridge or freezer.

Pumpkin Seed Meal: Having written a slew of recipes using nut meals, we got e-mails from readers with nut allergies, wanting an alternative. Pumpkin seed meal works as well as almond meal in baking. It's cheaper and higher in minerals too.

We know of no commercial source of pumpkin seed meal. No big deal, though; it's a snap to make your own. Raw, shelled pumpkin seeds are available at health food stores and at Mexican markets, where they're called *pepitas*. Dump the pumpkin seeds into your food processor and run it till they're the texture of coarse cornmeal. Store in an airtight container in the fridge or freezer.

Flaxseed Meal: Flaxseed is a true superfood. It's high in protein and fiber and is one of the best plant sources of omega-3 fatty acids. It's also high in lignans, an antioxidant that may protect against estrogenic forms of cancer, like breast cancer. All this, and it has a nice, mild, nutty flavor too.

Flaxseed is widely available but tough to grind. Fortunately, flaxseed meal is now widely distributed. Health food stores carry it, and many big grocery stores have it in the baking aisle. You can use Bob's Red Mill Golden Flaxseed Meal.

Store flaxseed meal in an airtight container or resealable plastic bag in the freezer. The healthy oils in it are perishable and degrade pretty rapidly once the seeds are ground, so the freezer is preferable to the fridge unless you're likely to use it up quite quickly.

Oat Bran: This is the outside coat of the oat grain. It's high in fiber, which lowers its glycemic load. We find oat bran useful in baked goods and also as a substitute for bread crumbs or crushed cereal in meat loaf and the like. You can find oat bran in the cereal aisle with the oatmeal.

Wheat Bran: The outside coat of the wheat grain. It's loaded with insoluble fiber, which helps keep your digestive tract healthy. Available at most grocery stores and all health food stores.

Wheat Germ: Wheat germ is the little bit inside a wheat kernel that would have actually become the plant. It's the part of the wheat kernel where most of the protein and vitamins are. I've included modest quantities of wheat germ in a couple of recipes to give them a grainy flavor without much starch. We recommend raw wheat germ, since you're going to cook it anyway. Raw wheat germ is available at health food stores and sometimes in the baking aisle of grocery stores. If you can't find it, go ahead and use the toasted wheat germ you find in the cereal aisle. Store wheat germ in the fridge.

Vege-Sal: Vege-Sal is a seasoned salt, but it's nothing like traditional "seasoned salt." Instead it's salt mixed with powdered, dried vegetables. The flavor is subtle, but we think it improves many recipes. In numerous recipes we've given you a choice of using Vege-Sal or salt. Widely available at health food stores.

Chili Garlic Paste: Also known as *chili garlic sauce,* this Southeast Asian condiment consists largely—as you would expect—of hot chile peppers and garlic. Once you have it in your refrigerator, you'll find hundreds of ways to use it. Look for chili garlic paste at Asian markets or the international foods aisle of big grocery stores. As long as it's refrigerated, chili garlic paste appears to keep nearly forever.

Low-Sugar Preserves: We prefer these, not only because they have less sugar than regular preserves but also because I think they taste better. We use Smucker's brand low-sugar preserves, but if you like, use whatever you have on hand.

Bouillon Concentrate: Bouillon concentrate adds flavor to many dishes. We like Better Than Bouillon jarred paste concentrate, because unlike many bouillon granules or cubes, it actually contains chicken or beef or ham or whatever flavor is listed on the label. If you can't find Better Than Bouillon, buy granules or liquid concentrate rather than cubes, which are more difficult to dissolve.

Fish Sauce: A traditional Southeast Asian condiment, also known as *nuoc mam* or *nam pla,* fish sauce is widely used in Thai and Vietnamese cooking. Look in the international aisle of your big grocery store or at an Asian market. Fish sauce doesn't go bad or need refrigeration.

Coconut Oil: Coconut oil has been shunned for the past few decades because it is very highly saturated. Turns out that despite—or possibly because of—that, coconut oil is very healthful stuff. It is rich in lauric acid, a fat that stimulates metabolism by improving thyroid function. Despite being saturated, lauric acid tends to lower "bad" cholesterol and raise "good" cholesterol. Medical studies in India, where coconut oil is a traditional cooking fat, found that when it was replaced by less-saturated oils, the rates of both heart disease and type 2 diabetes *increased*. Add to this that because of being very saturated, coconut oil does not turn rancid easily. Except for extra virgin coconut oil, which does have a pleasant coconut odor, coconut oil is quite bland. We use it often for frying and also as a substitute for trans fat–laden hydrogenated vegetable shortening. Coconut oil can be found at Asian markets and in the international aisle of big grocery stores.

Low-Carb Tortillas: These are more like flour tortillas than corn tortillas. Much of the flour is replaced with fiber and a little soy protein. We prefer La Tortilla Factory brand, because they're the highest in fiber—and therefore lowest in digestible, absorbable carbohydrate. Use them for quesadillas, wraps, breakfast burritos, even pizza crusts. If you can't find them in your hometown, you can order low-carb tortillas online. They keep pretty well, so order enough to last you for several weeks.

Canned Black Soybeans: Most beans are pretty starchy. They have a low enough glycemic load that you can eat them in moderation, but large doses may spike blood sugar, especially when they're mashed or pureed. Soybeans are the exception, and black soybeans are the least starchy of the bunch. Soybeans are a pain to cook at home; they take forever to get soft. But Eden brand canned black soybeans are available at health food stores and even in the health food section of some big grocery stores. They're awfully bland on their own, but they're good in chili and some soups. If you can't find black soybeans, any canned soybeans can be substituted.

Sucanat: Sucanat is sugarcane juice that has been dried and ground into a coarse powder. It tastes a lot like brown sugar, but it's not sticky like brown sugar. It has vitamins and minerals that brown sugar lacks. You can buy Sucanat at health food stores. If you can't find it, brown sugar will work, but it has no vitamins or minerals.

Some of you may be wary of all concentrated sugars, this one included. We have used Sucanat in developing these recipes, and I haven't noticed any ill effects, but we don't use it much in day-to-day cooking.

If you prefer not to use Sucanat, you may substitute brown sugar–flavored maltitol, which is available through online specialty merchants, or brown sugar Splenda blend, which combines Splenda with brown sugar. You can also substitute Splenda plus a little blackstrap molasses, but this will change the texture of your finished product a bit.

Splenda: Splenda is the sweetener we reach for most often. We think it tastes very good, it works in a wide range of applications, it doesn't lose sweetness when heated, and because it has the same degree of sweetness as sugar, it can be substituted one-for-one, making it easy to gauge how much to use. I have often given you the choice between using a little Splenda and using a little sugar.

Many recipes in this book offer you a choice between using Sucanat or sugar and using Splenda. In those recipes, the first sweetener listed is the sweetener analyzed for in the nutrition information.

14

Eggs and Dairy

Of all the nutritional slander of the low-fat era, none is so wrongheaded, so downright dangerous, as the demonizing of eggs. Please, please, do not be afraid of eggs. There is nothing more nutritious on the planet—or at your grocery store. Should you throw away the yolks? Only if you want to discard most of the vitamins, minerals, and antioxidants along with them.

It seemed intuitively obvious that eating cholesterol would cause high blood cholesterol, but the research doesn't back up the hypothesis. Even the American Heart Association has reluctantly admitted that eggs don't appear to increase heart disease risk factors. (Nor does eating high-cholesterol foods as a group.)

So eat eggs! Not just for breakfast, but anytime you want a quick, satisfying, and delicious meal. Eggs can be downright cheap, but I'd like to recommend that if they're available near you and your budget can accommodate them, you buy pastured eggs from small local farms. They're superior, in both flavor and nutrition.

If you can't find or afford pastured eggs, eggs from conventionally raised chickens are still a nutritional bargain. Buy them by the 18-egg carton. And a word to the wise: Kept refrigerated, eggs will be okay for omelets, casseroles, and boiling for at least

6 weeks. When they're a loss-leader sale item in the spring, buy as many cartons as you can fit in the refrigerator.

I'm going to assume you already know how to fry, scramble, or boil an egg and not take up space with recipes for those preparations. But they're all fine ways to cook eggs; enjoy them whenever you like.

Omelets

If I could teach everyone one cooking skill, it would be how to make an omelet. There is no other skill that allows you such a tremendous range of fast and fabulous meals. Too, when you first cut your glycemic load, it can seem odd to eat fried or scrambled eggs without toast on the side. But somehow an omelet seems like a complete meal all by itself.

Fortunately, making omelets is a whole lot easier than rumor would have you believe. Here's how:

Dr. Rob Says: Are You Really What You Eat?

A lot of people, even some doctors, take the old saying "You are what you eat" literally. They think that people get fat from eating fat and get high blood cholesterol from eating cholesterol. What they don't realize is that the human body can quickly convert carbs to fat, fat to carbs, and either to cholesterol. That potato you ate? Within a couple of hours, your body turns it to fat.

As for cholesterol, your liver makes about three times more than you eat. If you eat less, it just makes more. If you eat more, it just makes less. Don't blame your diet for high blood cholesterol. Blame your parents. It's mainly a genetic thing.

- You'll need the right pan—a 7" to 9" skillet with a good nonstick coating and sloping sides is ideal.
- Get prepared. Once you start making your omelet, things go very quickly, so have your omelet filling standing by. If you're using cooked vegetables, cook them first and have them standing by. If you're using cheese, grate or slice it ahead of time. If you're making an omelet to use up leftovers—a superb idea—warm them in the microwave oven first. Have a spatula by the stove too.
- Whether you're using a nonstick skillet or cooking spray, put your not-sticky skillet over medium-high heat. While it's heating, crack two eggs into a bowl and use a fork to scramble them. Unless the recipe says otherwise, don't add a thing—just mix up your eggs.
- When your skillet is hot, add a little oil or butter. Slosh it around to cover the bottom of the skillet.
- Drip one drop of the beaten eggs into the skillet. If it immediately sizzles and sets, your skillet is ready. (If the egg doesn't sizzle and set, let the skillet heat up a little more.) Dump in the beaten eggs all at once. Now comes the important part: *Don't just let your eggs sit there.* If you do, your eggs will be hopelessly overdone on the bottom before the top is set. An omelet is built up in layers.
- So grab that spatula you set by the stove. Start lifting the edges of cooked egg and letting the still-liquid egg run underneath. Do this all around the edge, using your other hand to tilt the skillet to let the raw egg run underneath. Within a minute or so, you won't have enough liquid egg left to run.
- Now turn your burner down to the lowest setting. (If you have an electric stove, it's a good idea to use two burners, the first on medium-high and a second on low, and switch burners.) Spread your filling over half of your disk of egg. Cover the skillet and let the omelet cook for a couple of minutes.
- Now take a peek. If the top surface is cooked and your cheese, if you're using any, is melted, it's done. If your omelet still looks underdone, cover it again and give it another minute or two.

Forget the Fat-Free Dairy Too

Plain yogurt is a good low-glycemic-load food that sticks to your ribs. Unfortunately, commercially sweetened yogurts are packed with sugar. Buy plain yogurt (don't bother with fat free), add some fruit, and sweeten to taste with a half teaspoon of sugar or artificial sweetener. Fruit and cottage cheese combine to make a quick low-glycemic-load standard that should keep you satisfied until lunch. Again, don't bother with the low-fat kind.

- When your omelet is done, slip your spatula under the naked side of your omelet and fold it over the filling. Lift the whole thing onto a plate and serve. (If you're making omelets for several people, have your oven on its lowest setting and keep the first ones warm in there as the later ones cook.)

That's it! It takes far less time to do than it's taken me to write this out. What to put in your omelet? All sorts of things. How about:

- Avocado slices and Monterey Jack, topped with salsa
- Sautéed mushrooms and onions
- Crumbled Italian sausage, cooked with peppers and onions, topped with pasta sauce
- Shredded mozzarella, topped with jarred pizza sauce
- Leftover chili, plus Cheddar cheese, topped with sour cream
- Leftover tuna salad, plus Swiss cheese
- Sliced ham and Swiss or Cheddar cheese, plus a smear of mustard
- Smoked salmon and cream cheese
- Raw spinach, crumbled feta, and chopped olives
- Sliced turkey and tomato, plus crumbled bacon
- Guacamole, tomatoes, and cheese

Almost anything that's good in a sandwich is good in an omelet, as are many dips. Once you get in the omelet habit, you'll find yourself looking at recipes and thinking, "Y'know, that combination would be good in an omelet."

Here are some great egg and dairy recipes to get you started. (While they are most often thought of as breakfast, you can make them for any meal of the day.)

Homemade Breakfast Burrito

Too busy to cook a hot breakfast? Make a batch of these fast-food favorites on Sunday, keep them in the refrigerator, and microwave them during the week before rushing off in the morning. They'll stick to your ribs all day. The trick is to reduce the glycemic load by using low-carb tortillas. The following recipe gives you the basics, but feel free to add fresh cilantro, sour cream, and lime juice.

> 6 ounces prepared pork sausage
> ¼ cup chopped onion
> ½ teaspoon chili powder
> 4 eggs
> 4 high-fiber, reduced-carb wheat tortillas
> 4 ounces cream cheese, cut into bits, or ½ cup grated
>   Cheddar cheese
> 1 medium tomato, seeded and chopped
> Salt and freshly ground black pepper to taste
> Salsa (optional)

1. Crumble the sausage into a skillet. Add the onion and chili powder. Mix together and cook over medium heat, stirring occasionally, until the meat is thoroughly cooked and the sausage and onion begin to brown, about 10 minutes. Transfer to a bowl and keep warm.

2. Scramble the eggs. Pour into the skillet used for cooking the sausage mixture. Cook, stirring frequently, just until the eggs are no longer runny, 2 to 4 minutes. Remove the pan from the heat.

3. Meanwhile, sprinkle each tortilla with a few drops of water, stack on a plate, and cover with a paper towel. Microwave on high for 30 seconds.

4. To assemble the burritos, lay the warm tortillas on serving plates. Divide the sausage mixture equally, making a band of filling across the middle of each tortilla. Top with equal portions of scrambled eggs, cheese, and tomato. Season with salt and pepper.

5. Fold one side of the tortilla over the filling, and then the other. Turn the burrito over to keep it closed. Garnish with salsa, if desired.

4 servings. Per serving: 448 calories, 21 g protein, 17 g carbohydrate, 33 g fat, 8 g fiber

Note: To make ahead of time, assemble each burrito with all the ingredients except the tomato, which is more difficult to keep fresh. Wrap the burritos in plastic wrap and refrigerate. To reheat, remove the plastic wrap and microwave each burrito on high for 1 minute. Serve topped with the fresh tomato.

Spinach-Mushroom Frittata

A frittata is an Italian omelet that doesn't need to be folded. This is a wonderful quick supper and a good choice if you have vegetarians over for dinner.

    2 tablespoons butter
    2 tablespoons olive oil
    1 large onion, chopped
    8 ounces sliced mushrooms
    1 clove garlic, crushed
    1 package (10 ounces) frozen chopped spinach, thawed
    6 large eggs
    ½ teaspoon ground black pepper
    ½ teaspoon salt
    2 teaspoons brown mustard
    1 teaspoon dried oregano
    ¾ cup grated fresh Parmesan cheese, divided
    ¾ cup grated fresh Romano cheese, divided

1. You'll need a big, heavy skillet with an ovenproof handle; I use my cast-iron skillet. Give it a shot of cooking spray and put it over medium heat. Add the butter and olive oil and swirl them together as the butter melts. Now add the onion and mushrooms and cook, stirring frequently.

2. When the mushrooms are soft and the onion is translucent, quite a lot of liquid will have cooked out of them. Stir in the garlic, turn the heat to low, and let the whole thing simmer for a couple more minutes while you drain the spinach. Do drain it well! The easiest way is to dump it into a strainer and press it hard with the back of a spoon. Then add the drained spinach to the mushrooms and onion and stir the whole thing together until everything is distributed evenly.

3. Break the eggs into a big bowl, preferably one with a pouring lip (a big measuring cup works well too), and add the pepper, salt, mustard, oregano, and ½ cup each of the Parmesan and Romano. Whisk together.

4. Pour the egg and cheese mixture over the veggies in the skillet. Spread everything into an even layer. Cover the skillet and cook over low heat for 12 to 15 minutes or until all but the very top is set. Turn on your broiler.

5. Sprinkle the reserved cheeses over the top. Now run the whole skillet under the broiler for 3 to 5 minutes, until the top is golden. Cut into wedges to serve.

6 servings. Per serving: 270 calories, 17 g protein, 7 g carbohydrate, 20 g fat, 2 g fiber

Zucchini-Pepper Frittata

My charming neighbors, Keith and Peter, grow more vegetables on their half-acre lot than you could possibly believe. I came up with this recipe when their zucchini were threatening to take over the neighborhood.

> 2 tablespoons olive oil
> 2 tablespoons butter
> 8 ounces zucchini, halved lengthwise and thinly sliced
> 1 medium yellow bell pepper, finely chopped
> 1 large onion, finely chopped
> 2 cloves garlic, crushed
> 1 cup finely chopped cooked chicken or turkey
> 8 eggs
> 2 tablespoons spicy brown mustard
> 1½ teaspoons Italian seasoning
> 3 tablespoons dry white wine
> 1½ cups shredded Muenster cheese, divided

1. Coat a heavy skillet with cooking spray and place over medium heat. Add the olive oil and butter. When the butter is melted, add the zucchini, bell pepper, onion, and garlic and cook, stirring frequently, until the onion is translucent and the zucchini and pepper have softened a bit. Stir in the chicken and turn to low heat.

2. Crack the eggs into a great big glass measuring cup or a mixing bowl. Add the mustard, Italian seasoning, wine, and 1 cup of the cheese. Whisk together.

3. Now pour the egg and cheese mixture over the veggies and chicken. Stir the whole thing just enough to make sure the egg mixture gets all the way to the bottom. Cover the skillet and let your frittata cook for 15 minutes. All except the very top should be set. Turn on your broiler.

4. Scatter the last ½ cup of cheese over the top. Now run the skillet under the broiler, about 8" away, for 5 minutes, or until the top is golden brown. Cut into wedges to serve.

6 servings. Per serving: 335 calories, 22 g protein, 6 g carbohydrate, 2 g fat, 1 g fiber

Colorful Herb Frittata

The orange carrot chunks, along with the green herbs, make for a festive dish. The carrot chunks add substance—replacing the starchy potato, which is a standard part of the usual frittata. This baked form of scrambled eggs takes well to so many different flavorings, from cooked ham, sausage, and smoked fish to mushrooms, sun-dried tomatoes, and cheese. Frittatas also keep well refrigerated, so you can eat a slice at a time over several days for a quick gourmet breakfast.

> 1 medium carrot, peeled and cut crosswise into 2" lengths
> 3 sprigs fresh dill
> 3 sprigs fresh parsley
> 2 scallions, trimmed
> 6 eggs
> 1 teaspoon Dijon mustard
> Salt to taste
> 2 tablespoons extra virgin olive oil
> Sour cream for garnish

1. Preheat the oven to 350°F.
2. Boil the carrot chunks in a small pot over medium-high heat until tender, about 10 minutes.
3. Meanwhile, remove the stems from the dill and parsley. Finely chop the 2 herbs. Slice the scallions crosswise into ¼"-thick pieces. Finely chop the carrots.
4. Break the eggs into a medium bowl and add the mustard. Beat the eggs with a fork. Mix the herbs, scallions, and carrots into the eggs. Season with salt.
5. Put the oil in a medium to large ovenproof skillet, preferably nonstick, over medium heat. When the oil is hot, pour the egg mixture into the skillet and reduce the heat to medium-low. Cook, undisturbed, until the bottom of the frittata is firm, about 7 minutes.
6. Transfer the skillet to the oven. Be careful not to grab the skillet handle when hot.

(continued)

7. Bake the frittata just until the top is no longer runny. Check for doneness after 10 minutes. Cook for another 5 minutes or so, but be very careful not to overcook.

8. Using an oven mitt, remove the skillet from the oven and place it on a work surface. Use a spatula to loosen the frittata from the pan. Tip the skillet and slide the frittata gently onto a serving platter. Serve immediately, or refrigerate to enjoy chilled. Garnish with sour cream.

6 servings. Per serving: 134 calories, 7 g protein, 4 g carbohydrate, 10 g fat, 1 g fiber

Apple, Cheddar, and Bacon Omelet

Apples and cheese are a classic combination, and so are cheese and bacon. Put all three together and—wow!

¼ **apple**
2 **teaspoons butter**
¼ **teaspoon Sucanat or Splenda**
2 **eggs**
¼ **cup (1 ounce) shredded sharp Cheddar cheese**
2 **slices bacon, cooked, drained, and crumbled, divided**

1. Trim the core out of the apple quarter and cut into 5 or 6 slices. Melt the butter in your skillet and add the apple slices. Cook, stirring frequently, over medium heat for 4 to 5 minutes, flip, and sprinkle with the Sucanat or Splenda. When the apple slices are soft and a little browned, remove from the skillet.

2. Give your skillet a squirt of cooking spray and put it back over medium-high heat. Beat the eggs with a fork and make your omelet according to the method at the beginning of the chapter. Put the cheese in first, then the apple slices and half the crumbled bacon. When you've folded and plated your omelet, top with the rest of the bacon and serve.

1 serving. Per serving: 406 calories, 22 g protein, 7 g carbohydrate, 32 g fat, 1 g fiber

Avocado, Bacon, and Spinach Omelets

This recipe is for two omelets because leftover avocado might turn brown in the fridge. If you want to halve this recipe, coat the cut side of your leftover avocado half with lime or lemon juice, drop it in a resealable plastic bag, seal it most of the way, then suck the air out before you finish sealing the bag. This will keep it from browning for a day or two.

> 4 eggs
> ½ cup (2 ounces) Monterey Jack cheese, sliced or
>   shredded
> ½ cup fresh baby spinach
> 1 avocado, pitted, peeled, and sliced
> 2 scallions, including the crisp part of the greens, sliced
> 4 slices bacon, cooked and drained

1. Assemble all the filling ingredients by the stove.

2. Make your omelets one at a time, according to the directions at the beginning of this chapter. Layer the first 2 beaten eggs with half the cheese, then half the spinach, avocado, and scallion.

3. Crumble 2 slices of bacon over that. When the omelet is folded and plated, put it in a warm spot or put a big pot lid over it while you repeat the process with the second half of the ingredients; then serve.

2 servings. Per serving: 478 calories, 24 g protein, 10 g carbohydrate, 39 g fat, 3 g fiber

Sort-of-Indian Omelet

This recipe is adapted from the wonderful Indian cookbook *5 Spices, 50 Dishes,* by Ruta Kahate. We haven't tried the authentic version, but this version's great. As you'll see, in this omelet you just mix the fillings right into the eggs.

> 2 eggs
> 2 tablespoons finely chopped onion
> 1 clove garlic, minced
> 1 tablespoon finely chopped tomato
> 1 tablespoon finely chopped fresh cilantro
> ⅛ teaspoon chili garlic paste
> Pinch of salt
> Pinch of ground turmeric
> 2 teaspoons coconut oil

1. Whisk the eggs, then stir in the onion, garlic, tomato, cilantro, chili garlic paste, salt, and turmeric.
2. Give your 9" skillet a squirt of cooking spray and put over medium-high heat. Add the oil; slosh it around as it melts to coat the bottom of the skillet and let it get hot.
3. Add the egg mixture and let it cook, without stirring, till the edges are set. Then start the process of lifting the edges and letting raw egg run underneath, keeping in mind that with all that yumminess in the beaten egg, it won't run as easily.
4. When there's not enough raw egg left to run underneath, carefully flip the omelet. It should be golden brown on the cooked side. Let the other side cook for a minute or so; then serve.

1 serving. Per serving: 225 calories, 12 g protein, 4 g carbohydrate, 18 g fat, 1 g fiber

Note: The book from which I adapted this recipe said that tomato ketchup was mandatory with this sort of omelet, but I think it's fine without. Do as you like.

Spring-in-the-Wintertime Scramble

If you're feeling too lazy to bother with an omelet, you can always just scramble wonderful tidbits into your eggs for a charmingly simple and fresh-tasting dish.

> 2 teaspoons butter
> ¾ cup sliced mushrooms
> 2 teaspoons finely chopped red onion
> ¾ cup frozen peas
> 3 eggs
> Salt and ground black pepper to taste

1. Give your medium skillet a shot of cooking spray and put it over medium-low heat. Drop in the butter and start cooking the mushrooms and onion, stirring frequently.

2. Meanwhile, put the peas in a small microwaveable dish, add a couple of teaspoons of water, cover, and microwave on high for just a minute.

3. When the mushrooms have changed color and softened, drain the peas and add them to the skillet. Stir them into the mushrooms and onion.

4. Now break your eggs into a dish and mix them up with a fork. Pour them into the skillet and scramble until set. Plate, add salt and pepper, and eat.

1 serving. Per serving: 363 calories, 23 g protein, 19 g carbohydrate, 21 g fat, 6 g fiber

Savory Scramble

Bacon and eggs, only more exciting.

> **2 teaspoons butter**
> **3 scallions, including the crisp greens, sliced**
> **3 eggs**
> **1 tablespoon half-and-half**
> **¾ teaspoon brown mustard**
> **⅛ teaspoon ground black pepper**
> **⅛ teaspoon salt**
> **3 slices bacon, cooked and drained, divided**
> **1 tablespoon chopped parsley**

1. Give your medium skillet a shot of cooking spray and put it over medium heat. Melt the butter and throw in the scallions.

2. While that's happening, use a fork to beat the eggs, half-and-half, mustard, pepper, and salt in a cereal bowl.

3. Crumble 2 of the 3 slices of cooked bacon into the egg mixture. Now pour it over the scallions and scramble the whole thing.

4. Put your eggs on a plate, crumble the last slice of bacon over them, and scatter the parsley over the whole dish. Then devour!

1 serving. Per serving: 414 calories, 24 g protein, 6 g carbohydrate, 32 g fat, 1 g fiber

Eggs Puttanesca

Puttanesca sauce is a wonderful pasta sauce loaded with olives, capers, and artichoke hearts. You can find it with the other pasta sauces in your grocery store. In this quick and easy but wonderful dish, you poach the eggs in this flavorful sauce.

> **1 cup puttanesca sauce**
> **4 eggs**
> **2 tablespoons grated fresh Parmesan cheese**

1. In a medium skillet, heat the puttanesca sauce over medium-low heat. When it's simmering, break the eggs into the skillet and cover. Poach for 5 to 7 minutes, or until the whites are set.

2. Transfer the eggs to 2 plates with a slotted spoon, then spoon the sauce remaining in the skillet over them. Top with Parmesan and serve immediately.

2 servings. Per serving: 221 calories, 15 g protein, 9 g carbohydrate, 14 g fat, 1 g fiber

Note: Try poaching eggs in other sauces as well, such as Creole sauce or salsa topped with Monterey Jack.

Breakfast Custard

You could have this for dessert, of course, but it has enough protein to serve as breakfast. How lovely would chilled lemon-vanilla custard be on a sultry summer morning? By the way, evaporated milk comes in 12-ounce cans and 5-ounce cans, so you want one of each.

> 2 cans (17 ounces) evaporated milk
> 4 large eggs
> ⅓ cup Splenda
> 1 teaspoon lemon extract
> ½ teaspoon vanilla extract
> 2 tablespoons vanilla whey protein powder
> Pinch of salt
> 1 teaspoon grated lemon peel

1. Preheat the oven to 325°F. Spray a 1-quart baking dish with cooking spray.
2. Whisk together the milk, eggs, Splenda, lemon extract, vanilla extract, whey protein powder, salt, and lemon peel. Pour into the prepared baking dish.
3. Place a baking pan larger than your baking dish in the oven. Put the baking dish in the center of it. Now pour water into the baking pan, as deep as you can without getting water into the baking dish.
4. Bake for 1½ hours, or until a knife inserted in the center comes out clean. Remove from the oven (it's safer to lift the baking dish out of the water bath and let the water cool before moving the baking pan) and let the custard cool. Then chill overnight before serving.

4 servings. Per serving: 284 calories, 20 g protein, 17 g carbohydrate, 15 g fat, trace fiber

Ham, Cheese, and Broccoli Egg Puff

You'll thank me for this the next time you have leftover ham in the house. And it reheats beautifully. Just cut a square and microwave on medium for a couple of minutes. Makes a great quick breakfast!

>   6 eggs
>   1 cup cottage cheese
>   2 teaspoons prepared horseradish
>   1½ teaspoons mustard powder
>   ¼ teaspoon salt or Vege-Sal
>   ¼ teaspoon ground black pepper
>   1½ cups small ham cubes
>   1 package (10 ounces) frozen chopped broccoli, thawed
>   and drained
>   2 cups shredded regular or reduced-fat Cheddar cheese

1. Preheat the oven to 325°F. Spray an 8" × 8" baking dish with cooking spray.

2. In a mixing bowl, whisk together the eggs, cottage cheese, horseradish, mustard powder, salt, and pepper.

3. Pour half the egg mixture into the prepared baking dish. Sprinkle the ham cubes in an even layer over the egg, then the broccoli in an even layer over that. Sprinkle the shredded cheese evenly over that, then pour the remaining egg mixture over the whole thing.

4. Bake for 50 to 60 minutes, or until puffed and turning golden. Cut into squares to serve.

9 servings. Per serving: 218 calories, 18 g protein, 4 g carbohydrate, 14 g fat, 1 g fiber

Salmon and Asparagus Casserole

What an elegant Sunday brunch! And it's just as good on Monday too if you have leftovers. Just cut a square and microwave on medium for a couple of minutes.

½ pound salmon fillet
1 pound thin asparagus spears
6 eggs
1 cup cottage cheese
1½ tablespoons lemon juice
½ teaspoon lemon pepper
½ teaspoon salt or Vege-Sal
2 teaspoons snipped fresh dill or ½ teaspoon dried
8 ounces Swiss cheese slices

1. Preheat the oven to 350°F. Spray an 8" × 8" baking dish with cooking spray.
2. If your salmon has skin, remove it. Now flake the salmon or chop it up. Reserve.
3. Snap the ends off the asparagus where it breaks naturally. Lay it on your cutting board and cut it into ½" lengths. Reserve.
4. In a mixing bowl, preferably one with a pouring lip, whisk together the eggs, cottage cheese, lemon juice, lemon pepper, salt or Vege-Sal, and dill. Pour half of this mixture into the prepared baking pan.
5. Sprinkle the flaked salmon evenly over the egg mixture. Layer the asparagus over that, then lay the cheese slices evenly on top. Pour the rest of the egg mixture over the whole thing.
6. Bake for 50 to 60 minutes, until puffed and golden. Cut into squares to serve.

9 servings. Per serving: 197 calories, 20 g protein, 4 g carbohydrate, 11 g fat, 1 g fiber

Breakfast Cereal Sundae

Commercial flavored yogurts are loaded with sugar to appeal to the palates of 14-year-olds. However, you can easily make your own with much less sugar, starting with unsweetened yogurt and adding flavorings like cinnamon, vanilla, strawberries, blueberries, mango, or fresh mint and sweetening to taste with a half teaspoon or so of sugar. You can also layer the yogurt with cereal and fruit. A nectarine was chosen for this recipe because these come to market sweet and juicy almost year-round and taste almost like peaches. Serve this concoction in an ice cream sundae glass or a large, stemmed wine or water glass, and you'll be starting the day with a nutritious, high-fiber dessert.

> **1 sprig mint**
> **½ cup yogurt**
> **½ cup All-Bran cereal**
> **1 ripe nectarine, sliced**
> **Berries for garnish (optional)**

1. Chop the mint leaves and put them in a small bowl along with the yogurt. Stir to combine.
2. Put one-third of the All-Bran into the bottom of an ice cream sundae glass. Top with one-third of the yogurt and a couple of nectarine slices.
3. Repeat this layering sequence twice, using up all the ingredients.
4. For your "cherry on top," top the sundae with a few raspberries or a strawberry, if desired, and sit down to breakfast.

1 serving. Per serving: 226 calories, 9 g protein, 45 g carbohydrate, 6 g fat, 13 g fiber

Strawberry Smoothie

Frozen fruit gives this the great frosty texture of a milkshake. Feel free to use any fruit—blueberries, blackberries, raspberries, frozen berry blend, frozen peach slices. You can freeze precut melon or pineapple chunks from the produce department to throw into smoothies. If you freeze bananas to use in your smoothies, cut them into a few chunks first to make them easier to blend.

> **1 cup plain yogurt**
> **½ cup milk**
> **½ cup unsweetened frozen strawberries**
> **2 tablespoons vanilla whey protein powder**
> **1 teaspoon to 2 tablespoons Splenda or stevia (which is a
>   lot sweeter than Splenda)**
> **Guar or xanthan (optional, but makes it thicker)**

Throw the yogurt, milk, strawberries, whey protein powder, Splenda or stevia, and guar or xanthan (if desired) into your blender and blend until smooth.

1 serving. Per serving: 375 calories, 34 g protein, 22 g carbohydrate, 14 g fat, 2 g fiber

Yogurt Parfait

This makes a great breakfast, but it's a yummy bedtime snack too.

> 1 teaspoon vanilla extract (or do what I do and use a
>   couple of capfuls)
> 1 tablespoon Splenda, or to taste
> 1 cup plain yogurt
> ½ cup fruit—berries are great, as are sliced peaches or
>   nectarines (use thawed unsweetened frozen fruit in
>   the winter)
> ¼ cup All-Bran, All-Bran Extra Fiber, or Fiber One cereal

1. Do you really need instructions? Stir the vanilla and Splenda into the yogurt and add the fruit. Sprinkle the All-Bran over the whole thing and eat.

2. Taking lunch to work? Stir up the vanilla yogurt in a snap-top container and throw in frozen fruit, without thawing it. Carry the All-Bran in a zip-top bag. The fruit will keep the yogurt cold for several hours. When lunch rolls around, just add the All-Bran to the yogurt and fruit and devour.

1 serving. Per serving: 231 calories, 11 g protein, 23 g carbohydrate, 9 g fat, 7 g fiber

The Fiber Secret

All-Bran is undoubtedly the best way of ensuring adequate insoluble fiber. The reason some people find bran cereal somewhat unsatisfying is probably that it doesn't contain enough fat and protein. Adding a handful of chopped walnuts corrects that problem and turns it into a hearty meal. You can also liven it up by eating it with yogurt instead of milk, throwing in a spoonful or two of some other kind of cereal, or adding some fruit.

15

Baked Goods and Other Grains

Perhaps the hardest part of getting used to the Glycemic Load Diet is learning to live without grains. We've been told so often, for so long, that grains are good for us, that bread is the staff of life. We can understand intellectually why it's not so, why grains are the worst thing for us. Yet somehow it still feels wrong to pass them up.

For so many of us, grains are comfort food. All our lives we've been eating cereal for breakfast, a sandwich for lunch, chicken noodle soup when we have a cold, Mom's homemade bread, hot out of the oven. It's disorienting to give these foods up.

You'll get over it; we promise. As your waistline shrinks, as you feel better and better, as your energy level skyrockets, as your health improves, you'll get over it.

Don't I Need Whole Grains?

In recent years we've been told that whole grains are incredibly beneficial, that the more of them we eat the healthier we'll be. But here's the thing: Those studies compare people who eat whole grains with people who eat refined grains—grains with the fiber,

Dr. Rob Says: Whole Grains = Sugar Rocks with a Few Vitamins

There's no doubt that whole grain bread and brown rice have more vitamins and fiber than white bread and white rice, but when it comes to raising your blood sugar, they're just as bad, even worse. Whole grains are packed solid with starch crystals. These little rocks turn to sugar as soon as they hit your digestive tract. Unless you're malnourished, you don't need the vitamins. There isn't enough fiber in them to do you any good. You certainly don't need the sugar shock.

vitamins, and minerals removed. We've yet to see one study that shows that people who eat lots of whole grains are healthier than people who don't eat grains at all.

Grains have been part of the human diet only since the Agricultural Revolution, about 10,000 years ago—a tiny fraction of our history. We all have hunter-gatherer ancestors—and hunter-gatherers don't eat grains. If grains were an essential part of human nutrition, our ancestors wouldn't have survived long enough to figure out farming and start eating them.

A Few Store-Bought Items

There are a few commercially made baked goods that fit into a low-glycemic-load diet. They manage this by having some of the starch replaced by fiber. Fiber is a carbohydrate, but you can't digest it, so it doesn't push up your blood sugar or trigger an insulin release.

- **Low-carb tortillas.** A great thing to keep on hand.
- **Low-carb bread.** True low-carb bread is getting harder and harder to find, but there are still a few brands out there. Read labels. At this writing, Trader Joe's carries

low-carb whole grain bread, Arnold Bakery lists a "carb-counting" bread on its Web site, and Healthy Life bakery lists a few varieties that have 6 grams of nonfiber carbohydrate per slice. Our favorite low-carb bread has long been the Carb Conscious bread from Natural Ovens Bakery of Manitowoc, Wisconsin; I've been ordering it from their Web site, naturalovens.com.

- **Fiber crackers.** Most crackers have not only a high glycemic load but trans fats as well. Bad stuff. But there are two brands of crackers we know of that are mostly wheat bran: Bran-a-Crisp and Fiber Rich. We haven't noticed a difference between the two; buy whichever you can find or find cheaper. Fiber crackers are pretty boring on their own, but they make an agreeably crunchy base for cheese, liverwurst, pâté, or tuna salad.

- **All-Bran, All-Bran Extra Fiber, and Fiber One.** These are the only cereals we know of that have a low glycemic load. If you choose one of these for breakfast, eat a protein food with it. These cereals also are good for making crumb crusts (page 319) and yogurt parfaits (page 168).

Diluting the Starch

The trick to creating baked goods and other grain products with a low glycemic load is to dilute the starch with a combination of fiber, protein, and fat. These recipes use bran, ground seeds and nuts, and protein powders to replace much of the flour. We've left just enough grain to get the familiar flavor and texture.

This means that this chapter, more than any other chapter in the book, will require you to lay in a stash of specialty ingredients. Your best bet for finding them all will be a good health food store.

About Baking Your Own Low-Carb Bread

We were torn about bread recipes. We believe we've figured out the solution. Here it is: When you make these recipes in your bread machine, do not simply put the ingredients in your bread machine, turn it on, and walk away. Instead, turn on the machine and let it knead the dough for 3 to 4 minutes. Then open the lid and look at your dough ball.

How does it look? Is it sticking to the sides of the bread case and "puddling" at the bottom? It's too wet. Add more of the dry ingredients (vital wheat gluten, flour, bran, protein powder) 1 tablespoon at a time. Sprinkle a tablespoon of one of those dry ingredients over the dough ball and let the machine knead it in before you decide whether you need more. If you do, add a little of the next dry ingredient—you'll be keeping your proportions right. When the dough forms a cohesive ball, it's right, and you can close the machine and walk away.

If you look at your dough ball and it's breaking into a couple of lumps instead of forming one ball, or if it's leaving dry flour behind, your dough is too dry. Sprinkle 1 tablespoon of water over the dough ball and let the machine knead it in. Repeat until you have a single cohesive ball that picks up all the flour. Then you can close the machine and walk away.

It's also good to know that the online low-carb stores carry low-carb bread machine mixes. A quick Web search will turn them up.

And Remember . . .

These baked-good recipes have a low glycemic load only if you eat them in moderation—1 serving a day, no more. (That's 1 serving a day of one of these, not one of each!) Glycemic load equals glycemic index times total grams of carbohydrate. Eat too many grams of carbohydrate, even from these recipes, and you'll wind up with a high glycemic load.

High-Fiber Bran Muffins

Most commercial bran muffins fall short when it comes to fiber, and because of their high flour content, they have unacceptable glycemic loads. However, you can make your own power-packed bran muffins with enough fiber to do you some good. You can reduce the glycemic load by mixing almond meal with whole wheat flour. For variety, you can add apple chunks, blueberries, or cranberries; substitute walnut oil for some of the safflower oil; use toasted almonds or walnuts; or spice with grated fresh ginger. These handy muffins deliver more than 10 grams of fiber each, as much as a bowl of All-Bran cereal.

> 1½ cups All-Bran cereal
> 1 cup whole almonds or whole wheat flour
> 3 cups wheat bran
> 3 tablespoons whole wheat flour (if using almond meal)
> ⅓ cup dark brown sugar
> 1 teaspoon baking powder
> 1 teaspoon baking soda
> 2 teaspoons ground allspice
> 1 teaspoon ground cinnamon
> ½ teaspoon ground nutmeg
> ½ teaspoon salt
> ½ cup apple chunks, blueberries, cranberries, or nuts
>   (optional)
> 3 eggs
> 1¼ cups milk
> ½ cup unrefined safflower oil
> 1 teaspoon vanilla extract
> Butter for greasing muffin cups

1. Adjust the oven rack to the lower-middle position. Preheat the oven to 350°F.

2. In a food processor with a metal blade, process the All-Bran until it has the texture of bread crumbs. Transfer to a large bowl. If using almonds instead of flour, process the almonds until they have the texture of cornmeal.

(continued)

3. Add the almonds or flour to the bowl, along with the wheat bran, flour (if using almond meal), sugar, baking powder, baking soda, allspice, cinnamon, nutmeg, and salt. Stir to combine the ingredients. Add the fruit or nuts, if desired.

4. Break the eggs into another large bowl and lightly beat with a fork. Add the milk, oil, and vanilla extract. Whisk to combine thoroughly.

5. Add about one-third of the dry ingredients to the egg-milk mixture and mix thoroughly. Repeat until all the ingredients are used.

6. Coat the cups of a 12-cup muffin pan lightly with butter. Spoon the batter into the muffin cups, filling them to the rim. Bake until a wooden pick inserted into the center of one of the muffins comes out clean or with a few moist particles adhering to it, about 20 minutes. Remove from the oven and cool slightly on a rack, about 5 minutes. Remove the muffins from the tin and serve warm.

12 muffins. Per muffin: 231 calories, 8 g protein, 27 g carbohydrate, 14 g fat, 11 g fiber

Cinnamon, Flax, and Bran Granola

We hear from many people who have a little problem with, er, regularity when they first drop the grains from their diets. So we came up with recipes to help them get bran and other fiber. This granola will do just that. It'll also keep you full and happy all morning long!

½ cup rolled oats
1 cup wheat bran
2 cups flaxseed meal
¾ cup wheat germ
½ cup shredded coconut meat
¾ cup oat bran
¼ cup vanilla whey protein powder
1½ teaspoons ground cinnamon
⅓ cup Splenda
⅛ cup Sucanat
¾ teaspoon salt
½ cup coconut oil, melted
¼ cup sugar-free pancake syrup or real maple syrup
2 tablespoons water
1½ teaspoons vanilla extract
½ cup chopped almonds
½ cup chopped pecans
½ cup chopped walnuts
½ cup shelled pumpkin seeds
½ cup sunflower seeds

1. Preheat the oven to 300°F. Line a big roasting pan with foil.
2. The easiest way to do this first part is with an electric mixer. Put the rolled oats, wheat bran, flaxseed meal, wheat germ, coconut, oat bran, whey protein powder, cinnamon, Splenda, Sucanat, and salt in a big bowl, and use the mixer to blend until all the ingredients are distributed evenly.
3. Mix the melted coconut oil with the syrup, water, and vanilla extract.

(continued)

4. Turn on your mixer and use it to slowly blend the liquid stuff into the dry stuff. Make sure everything is moistened evenly. Dump this mixture into your foil-lined roasting pan and use clean hands to press it out into an even layer. You want to compact it pretty well.

5. Slide the pan into the oven and bake for 30 minutes. Pull out the pan and set it on a heatproof surface (like the top of your stove). Use a pizza cutter or a knife to cut the baked stuff into squares about ½" across. Stir the whole mass around, then spread it into a layer again. (You're not packing it down this time.) Spread the nuts and seeds on top and slide the pan back into the oven.

6. Continue roasting the granola for at least another 45 minutes, stirring it every 15 to 20 minutes. You want to make sure the flax mixture is dried thoroughly. When it's done, pull it out, let it cool, and store it in an airtight container.

7. Eat like any granola—serve it with milk or cream, stir it into yogurt, however you like.

18 servings (½ **cup each**). Per serving: 350 calories, 15 g protein, 23 g carbohydrate, 26 g fat, 13 g fiber

Hot "Cereal"

On a chilly winter morning, you'll thank us for this recipe. Not only does this have a low glycemic load, but it has more protein than three eggs. It'll keep you going for hours!

½ cup flaxseed meal
½ cup almond meal
½ cup vanilla whey protein powder
¼ cup wheat bran
¼ cup oat bran
¼ teaspoon salt

1. Mix together the flaxseed meal, almond meal, whey protein powder, wheat bran, oat bran, and salt and store in an airtight container in your fridge or freezer.

2. To prepare the cereal, place ⅓ cup of the mixture in a bowl and stir in ⅓ cup of hot water. Let the mixture stand for a minute or so to thicken, then add milk or cream and the sweetener of your choice to taste. A little cinnamon is good too.

6 servings. Per serving: 227 calories, 25 g protein, 15 g carbohydrate, 11 g fat, 8 g fiber

Flax Pancakes

These pancakes passed the acid test: Family members scarfed them down with no "This tastes funny!" arguments. All this, and each pancake has more protein than three eggs and nearly twice the fiber of a bowl of oatmeal, with only 4 grams of nonfiber carbohydrate.

> **1 cup flaxseed meal**
> **1 cup vanilla whey protein powder**
> **¾ teaspoon baking soda**
> **1 tablespoon Splenda or Sucanat**
> **½ teaspoon salt**
> **¼ cup oat flour (you can leave this out if you want a truly grain-free pancake)**
> **1 teaspoon ground cinnamon**
> **1 cup plain yogurt**
> **2 eggs**

1. In a mixing bowl, combine the flaxseed meal, whey protein powder, baking soda, Splenda or Sucanat, salt, flour (if desired), and cinnamon and stir well to combine.

2. Spray your biggest skillet (or a griddle) with cooking spray and put it over medium-high heat. (If your skillet or griddle has a good nonstick surface, you can skip the cooking spray.)

3. While the pan is heating, whisk the yogurt and eggs into the dry ingredients, making sure there are no pockets of dry stuff left.

4. When your skillet is hot enough that a drop of water will skitter across the surface, it's time to cook. Scoop the batter with a ¼-cup measure. Fry the first side until the edges look dry, then flip the pancake and cook the other side.

5. Serve with the topping of your choice; I like low-sugar jelly.

12 pancakes. Per pancake: 208 calories, 21 g protein, 11 g carbohydrate, 10 g fat, 7 g fiber

Note: You can find whole grain oat flour at your health food store, or possibly in the baking aisle of your grocery store. In a pinch, run rolled oats through your food processor until they're finely ground.

Native American Flapjacks

Both corn and pumpkins are true American foods. These have enough cornmeal to give that great cornbread taste, with the protein and mineral kick from the pumpkin seeds.

⅔ cup whole grain cornmeal
⅔ cup hulled pumpkin seeds (pepitas), ground
1 teaspoon salt
½ teaspoon baking soda
¼ cup vanilla whey protein powder
3 tablespoons butter, melted
2 cups plain yogurt
2 eggs

1. Combine the cornmeal, ground pumpkin seeds, salt, baking soda, and whey protein powder in a mixing bowl. Stir them together until everything is distributed evenly.

2. In another bowl, whisk together the melted butter, yogurt, and eggs.

3. Put a big skillet or griddle, preferably with a nonstick coating, over medium-high heat. (If it doesn't have a nonstick coating, coat it well with cooking spray and add a little butter or oil between batches of cakes.) Let it get good and hot before you continue. Before you start cooking, your pan or griddle needs to be hot enough that a drop of water sprinkled on it skitters around the surface.

4. Dump the yogurt-egg mixture into the dry ingredients and stir together with a few swift strokes of your whisk—you want to stir just enough to make sure there are no pockets of dry stuff left.

5. Scoop 2 tablespoons of batter into the skillet (you can use a ⅛-cup measuring cup). Let each flapjack cook until the top surface looks dry before you flip it carefully. Let the other side brown, then serve with low-sugar jelly or sugar-free pancake syrup.

24 flapjacks. Per flapjack: 60 calories, 4 g protein, 4 g carbohydrate, 3 g fat, 1 g fiber

Apple-Walnut Pancakes

These make a terrific weekend breakfast, and each pancake has as much protein as three eggs! Refrigerate the leftovers and warm them up for breakfast the rest of the week.

½ cup flaxseed meal
¾ cup vanilla whey protein powder
¼ cup Splenda
1¼ teaspoons baking powder
¼ teaspoon baking soda
1 teaspoon ground cinnamon
⅛ teaspoon ground allspice
¼ teaspoon ground nutmeg
⅛ teaspoon salt
2 small Granny Smith apples
1½ cups milk
2 eggs
3 tablespoons butter, melted
½ teaspoon blackstrap molasses
½ cup chopped walnuts

1. In a mixing bowl, stir together the flaxseed meal, whey protein powder, Splenda, baking powder, baking soda, cinnamon, allspice, nutmeg, and salt.

2. Quarter the apples, cut the cores out, and whack each quarter in half. Using your food processor with the S blade in place, chop one of the apples pretty fine. Now add the second apple and continue chopping until that one is chopped fairly fine and the first one is even finer. (If you don't have a food processor, you could finely chop one apple and grate the other.)

3. Pour the milk into another bowl. Stir the eggs, melted butter, and molasses into it. At this juncture, put your biggest skillet or griddle over medium-high heat. If it doesn't have a nonstick surface, give it a coating of cooking spray.

4. Now dump the wet stuff into the dry stuff and whisk just until you're sure there are no pockets of dry stuff left. Whisk in the chopped apples and walnuts.

5. When your skillet or griddle is hot, scoop the batter with a ⅓-cup measure. Cook until the edges are dry and the surface is losing its shiny look. Serve with butter. If you like, you can sprinkle a little cinnamon and Splenda on top, but it's really not essential.

10 pancakes. Per pancake: 242 calories, 20 g protein, 12 g carbohydrate, 14 g fat, 5 g fiber

Sunflower-Cornmeal Cheese Crackers

These make a great snack, and they'd be killer with a bowl of chili or the Seriously Simple Southwestern Sausage Soup (page 255).

> 1 cup hulled sunflower seeds
> ⅓ cup whole grain cornmeal
> ½ teaspoon ground cumin
> ¼ teaspoon ground red pepper
> ¼ teaspoon salt
> 2 cups shredded Cheddar cheese
> 2 tablespoons water

1. Preheat the oven to 350°F.

2. In your food processor, using the S blade, grind the sunflower seeds to a fine meal. Add the cornmeal, cumin, ground red pepper, and salt. Pulse to mix.

3. Turn the processor on and feed the cheese in, bit by bit. When it's all in, dribble in the water. Then stop the processor.

4. Line a baking sheet with baking parchment. (Do not skip the parchment. You have been warned.) Turn the dough out onto the parchment—it will be crumbly but will stick together when you press it. Put another sheet of parchment over the dough. Using your hands and a rolling pin, coax the dough out to a thin, even, unbroken sheet—it should cover most of the baking sheet. Peel off the top sheet of parchment.

5. Now use a knife with a sharp, thin blade to score the dough into squares the size of Wheat Thins. Bake for 18 minutes and check. They should be browning a bit. If not, give them a few more minutes.

6. When your crackers come out of the oven, rescore them right away—they'll have melted together a bit. If the ones in the middle are still underdone, you can always transfer the ones that are done to an airtight container and give the ones that are still soft another run in the oven. If they're underdone, they won't be crisp.

4 dozen crackers. Per cracker: 39 calories, 2 g protein, 1 g carbohydrate, 3 g fat, trace fiber

16

Snacks and Other Pickup Food

"What can I have for a snack?" The question is a sign of our processed-food-eating times. To our great-grandparents, a snack was an apple, half a sandwich, the left-over drumstick from last night's chicken. But 21st-century Americans have been taught that a "snack" is something crunchy, salty, and usually starchy that comes out of a cellophane bag. (Starchy snacks are always salty. Why? Because without salt, starch is flavorless, of course.)

We've developed the habit of eating mindlessly for entertainment. How many times have you gone through a big bag of chips without thinking about it? I call it "the hand-to-mouth routine." There's a very simple reason we can do this: Starchy stuff doesn't fill you up. You can eat it nearly forever without feeling nauseated.

Welcome to Low-Glycemic-Load Snacking

Low-glycemic-load snacks are different: They're satisfying. This can require some retraining. Pay attention to your hunger. When you're actually hungry, eat. When you're full, stop. And don't eat again till you're hungry again. If you're bored, do something!

Here are some quick and easy snack ideas.

- **Fresh fruit of any kind.** Grab an apple, an orange, a plum, a peach—whatever's at hand. Most convenience stores have an apple or a banana somewhere.
- **Nuts.** Peanuts, mixed nuts, cashews, smoky-flavored almonds, all nuts are nutritious, healthful—and filling! They are also available at convenience stores and minimarts.
- **Pumpkin seeds.** My favorite crunchy, salty snack! Most minimarts have pumpkin seeds, salted in the shell. They're full of minerals, especially zinc. And the shells mean you have to eat them one by one, so one little bag lasts a long time.
- **Sunflower seeds.** A real nutritional powerhouse, sunflower seeds are available everywhere. If you crave variety, they come in interesting flavors like nacho cheese, ranch, and barbecue. As with pumpkin seeds, if you buy sunflower seeds in the shell, you can snack on them for a long time, because you'll have to crack and eat them one by one.
- **Pork rinds.** Despite their reputation as the nadir of junk food, pork rinds have twice as much protein as fat. Very filling!
- **Yogurt.** There's a wide variety of flavored yogurts in your grocer's dairy case, many sweetened with Splenda. Or spoon plain yogurt into a dish with cut-up fruit.
- **String cheese or other individually wrapped cheese bites.** An ounce or two of cheese will fill you up for hours.
- **Hard-cooked eggs.** Like cheese, hard-cooked eggs will keep you satisfied for a long time.
- **Beef jerky.** Available at truck stops and convenience stores everywhere.
- **Fiber crackers.** Most crackers have a high glycemic load and are full of trans fats to boot. But if you look around, you can find fiber crackers, the only crackers we know of with a really low glycemic load. The two brands we see most often are Fiber Rich and Bran-a-Crisp, which we find at health food stores. These crackers consist largely of bran, glued together with a modest quantity of rye flour. Fiber crackers are pretty boring on their own, but with a little

butter, peanut butter, or, my favorite, liverwurst, they're pretty good! Good with dips too.

- **Finn Crisp or Wasa Fiber Rye.** If you can't find fiber crackers, look for Finn Crisp or Wasa Fiber Rye. These flatbreads are crunchy and tasty and high in fiber. If you can limit yourself to just one or two, they shouldn't mess up your blood sugar.

The following recipes are great party foods, but you owe it to yourself to make them just for you and your family. Turn to them anytime you want something delicious you can simply pick up and shove in your face.

Sweet and Spicy Punks

These are addictive! Luckily, they're also good for you.

>   1 egg white
>   ⅓ cup Splenda or sugar
>   1 tablespoon chili powder
>   1 teaspoon ground cinnamon
>   ½ teaspoon salt
>   ¼ teaspoon ground cumin
>   ¼ teaspoon ground red pepper, or to taste
>   2 cups hulled pumpkin seeds (pepitas)

1. Preheat the oven to 350°F. Line a jelly roll pan or roasting pan with baking parchment.

2. Separate the egg white from the yolk. In a medium, fairly deep mixing bowl, whisk the white until it's frothy, but not whipped stiff.

3. Now whisk in the Splenda or sugar, chili powder, cinnamon, salt, cumin, and red pepper. Add half of the pumpkin seeds and stir until they're coated. Add the second cup and stir again, until they're all evenly coated.

4. Spread the pumpkin seeds evenly on the parchment-lined pan. Put them in the oven and set your timer for 5 minutes. When it goes off, stir the seeds, breaking any clumps apart as you do so. Put them back in and set the timer for another 5 minutes. Stir and separate again. Roast for a final 5 minutes, or until the seeds are dry and browning a bit.

5. Pull the seeds out of the oven, break up any clumps that are left, and let cool. Store in an airtight container if you don't devour them all that day.

8 servings. Per serving: 197 calories, 9 g protein, 8 g carbohydrate, 16 g fat, 2 g fiber

Spiced Peanuts

These subtly spicy-sweet, Indian-inspired peanuts are very, very special.

    2 tablespoons coconut oil
    2 tablespoons ground coriander
    1 tablespoon ground cumin
    2 tablespoons Sucanat
    2 teaspoons salt
    6 cups unsalted dry roasted peanuts
    1 tablespoon dark sesame oil

1. Preheat the oven to 350°F. Put the coconut oil in a big roasting pan and put it in the oven while it heats. Meanwhile, stir together the coriander, cumin, Sucanat, and salt.

2. Now pull out your roasting pan; the coconut oil will have melted. Dump your peanuts into the pan, add the sesame oil, and stir until the peanuts are coated evenly with the oils.

3. Sprinkle the seasoning mixture over the peanuts and stir until the peanuts are coated evenly.

4. Put the pan back in the oven and roast for 10 minutes, stir again, and roast for another 5 to 10 minutes.

24 servings. Per serving: 235 calories, 9 g protein, 9 g carbohydrate, 20 g fat, 3 g fiber

Note: Most grocery stores carry jars of unsalted dry roasted peanuts, but I get mine far cheaper in bulk at my health food store.

Five-Spice Wings

Five-spice powder is a traditional Chinese spice blend. Find it in the international aisle of your grocery store. These are sweet and spicy!

1 tablespoon five-spice powder
1 tablespoon Sucanat
½ teaspoon garlic powder
1½ teaspoons salt or Vege-Sal
4 pounds chicken wings
2 tablespoons tomato sauce
2 tablespoons low-sugar apricot preserves
¼ cup chicken broth
2 tablespoons Splenda
2 teaspoons soy sauce
2 tablespoons apple cider vinegar
1 teaspoon grated fresh ginger
2 tablespoons peanut oil or olive oil

1. Preheat the oven to 375°F.

2. Mix together the five-spice powder, Sucanat, garlic powder, and salt or Vege-Sal. Set aside 1 tablespoon of this mixture in a medium bowl. Sprinkle the rest evenly all over the wings. Lay the wings in a big roasting pan, skin side up, and slide them into the oven.

3. Grab that bowl with the set-aside seasoning mixture. Add the tomato sauce, preserves, broth, Splenda, soy sauce, vinegar, ginger, and oil and stir.

4. When the wings have been roasting for 15 to 20 minutes, baste them with the sauce you've made. Repeat about 15 minutes later and 15 minutes after that. By then your wings should be looking pretty done.

5. Serve the wings with the rest of the sauce for dipping.

8 servings. Per serving: 184 calories, 13 g protein, 4 g carbohydrate, 12 g fat, trace fiber

Huevos el Diablo

Or, if you prefer, Mexican Deviled Eggs, though they were invented in Indiana.

> 6 hard-cooked eggs
> 2 tablespoons canned chopped green chile peppers
> 2 tablespoons mayonnaise
> 1 tablespoon sour cream
> ¼ teaspoon ground cumin
> ½ teaspoon chili powder
> Pinch of ground red pepper, plus extra for garnish
> 2 tablespoons finely chopped red onion
> 2 tablespoons finely chopped fresh cilantro

1. Peel the eggs and split each one lengthwise. Turn the yolks out into a mixing bowl and put the whites on a plate.

2. Using a fork, mash the yolks as finely as you can. Then add the chile peppers, mayonnaise, and sour cream and mash again; you're trying to get the yolk mixture as creamy as you can.

3. Stir in the cumin, chili powder, and ground red pepper, mixing well to get the seasonings well distributed. Now add the onion and cilantro and stir again.

4. Stuff the yolk mixture back into the hollows of the whites. (If you really want to get fancy, you can use a pastry bag to pipe the yolk mixture in pretty rosettes, but I sure wouldn't bother.) Sprinkle a teeny bit of ground red pepper over the stuffed eggs for garnish and serve.

12 servings. Per serving: 60 calories, 3 g protein, 1 g carbohydrate, 5 g fat, trace fiber

Christmas Party Stuffed Eggs

What with the red bell peppers and the green parsley, these look as festive as they taste. But don't take the name too literally; they'll be welcome any time of year.

>   6 hard-cooked eggs
>   ¼ cup light mayonnaise
>   1½ teaspoons lemon juice
>   ½ teaspoon chicken bouillon concentrate
>   3 slices cooked bacon, finely crumbled
>   ⅛ teaspoon ground black pepper
>   2 dashes hot-pepper sauce
>   ⅛ teaspoon soy sauce
>   1½ teaspoons finely chopped scallion
>   1½ teaspoons finely chopped roasted red pepper, jarred
>   in water, drained
>   1½ teaspoons finely chopped parsley
>   Paprika (optional)

1. Peel the eggs, slice them in half lengthwise, and turn the yolks into a mixing bowl. Put the whites on a plate and set aside.

2. Mash the yolks thoroughly with a fork. Add the mayonnaise, lemon juice, and bouillon concentrate and mash again, stirring well, until the yolks are creamy and the bouillon concentrate is completely dissolved.

3. Now stir in the bacon, black pepper, hot-pepper sauce, soy sauce, scallion, roasted red pepper, and parsley. Stuff the yolk mixture back into the whites. Garnish with a sprinkle of paprika if you really want to, but they're pretty and very flavorful without it.

12 servings. Per serving: 60 calories, 4 g protein, 1 g carbohydrate, 4 g fat, trace fiber

Mustard-Horseradish Beef Roll-Ups

Easy and pretty.

>3 tablespoons mayonnaise
>3 tablespoons brown mustard
>1 tablespoon prepared horseradish
>1 scallion, finely chopped
>1 roasted red pepper, jarred in water, drained
>8 ounces deli roast beef, sliced medium-thick
>1½ cups (6 ounces) shredded Monterey Jack cheese

1. Mix together the mayonnaise, mustard, horseradish, and scallion. Slice the roasted red pepper lengthwise into as many strips as you have slices of beef.

2. Lay a slice of roast beef on your cutting board. Spread it with the mustard-mayo mixture and sprinkle it all over with shredded cheese. Now lay a strip of roasted red pepper across one end of the whole thing and roll up your slice of roast beef around it. Place on a plate, seam side down. Repeat until you're out of everything.

3. Chill your beef rolls for several hours. Right before serving, cut each across into 5 or 6 rolls about 1" long. Pierce them with wooden picks, arrange them prettily on a lettuce-lined plate, and serve.

24 servings. Per serving: 58 calories, 5 g protein, 1 g carbohydrate, 4 g fat, trace fiber

17

Salads

Salads don't have to be low-calorie rabbit food. Greens and oils complement rich ingredients like meat, cheese, nuts, avocados, and olives beautifully, and the glycemic loads of most salads are negligible. When you start a meal with a salad, the fiber slows the absorption of whatever glucose you get in the rest of your food. And there's no law that says salads have to fit on a small plate. You can make a meal of a hearty salad. In addition to the great salad recipes in the following pages, here are some popular low-glycemic-load salads you'll often find in cookbooks and restaurant menus.

- **Cobb salad:** This American classic combines romaine or any leaf lettuce with cubes of cooked chicken, tomato, bacon, crumbled blue cheese, avocado, and chopped egg. It's usually served with a vinaigrette or blue cheese dressing.
- **Taco salad:** This Tex-Mex favorite is simply taco fillings on a plate. Lettuce, tomato, avocado, and onion are combined with shredded beef or chicken flavored with taco seasoning and topped with shredded Cheddar cheese, salsa, and a dollop of sour cream.
- **Chopped salad:** The ingredients of this salad are finely chopped to the same size to blend their tastes. It includes

Dressing 101

Be wary of fat-free bottled dressings. Many of them replace oil with corn syrup, which makes them sugary liquids! Furthermore, studies show that if you eat salad without fat, you don't absorb the antioxidants. Stick with oil-based dressings, and they're even better if you make them yourself.

The basic proportions for a vinaigrette dressing are 2 to 3 parts olive oil to 1 part vinegar, lemon juice, or a combination of the two. You can add a clove of garlic to this, or a squirt of mustard, a dash of oregano or Italian seasoning, a pinch of sugar or Splenda, or a few drops of hot sauce. Of course, a little salt and ground black pepper is good. If you want a creamy dressing, add a dollop of mayonnaise. The variations are infinite, but the basics are unchanging.

Unless your family has violently differing opinions on salad dressings, do toss your salad with the dressing instead of simply pouring it on top of individual servings. It really improves the final product. Toss the salad with the dressing right before serving, or it will become soggy.

romaine lettuce, tomatoes, green peppers, and scallions paired with finely chopped Italian salami, mozzarella cheese, smoked turkey, and chickpeas and thoroughly tossed with vinaigrette dressing.

- **Tomato and mozzarella salad:** The Italians call this salad *caprese,* and it consists of slices of tomato topped with slices of fresh mozzarella, sprinkled with slivers of fresh basil, and drizzled with olive oil—a special treat in the summertime, when delicious tomatoes and fresh basil are available.

- **Greek salad:** This tasty classic salad includes tomato; cucumber; onion; marinated artichoke hearts; kalamata olives; sometimes lettuce, sometimes not; and chunks of feta cheese tossed with olive oil.
- **Caesar salad:** This one needs no introduction; it has become so popular that you'll find it on most menus. Combine romaine lettuce, Caesar dressing with or without anchovies, and shredded Parmesan cheese, and if you like, top with shrimp or chicken.

Salad Niçoise

Instead of potato, this version of the classic niçoise uses an array of complementary flavors including, if desired, a piquant onion relish (see page 197). It comes together as an arranged plate of colorful vegetables with reds, yellows, greens, and rosy purple. Serve it with ripe Brie or Camembert or, for variety, make it with fresh tuna steak or salmon.

½ pound fresh green beans, trimmed
2 eggs
2 cans (6 ounces each) tuna, packed in water, drained
1 bell pepper, preferably yellow or red
4 cups romaine lettuce, chopped into thin strips
2 tablespoons chopped fresh basil
1 tablespoon capers
6 tablespoons extra virgin olive oil
2 tablespoons balsamic vinegar
1 teaspoon Dijon mustard
Salt and ground black pepper to taste
8 cherry tomatoes, halved
8 olives, preferably niçoise or kalamata
Molly's Piquant Onion Relish (page 197), optional
8 anchovies

1. Steam the green beans for 10 minutes until al dente and still bright green.
2. Boil the eggs for 10 to 12 minutes, so the yolks are pleasantly creamy, or 15 minutes if you want them cooked through. Plunge the eggs into cold running water for 2 minutes and gently remove the peel. Quarter the eggs and set them aside.
3. Put the tuna, bell pepper, romaine, basil, and capers in a large bowl and toss to combine.
4. To make the dressing, put the oil in a small bowl and add the vinegar, mustard, salt, and black pepper. Stir vigorously and pour over the tuna mixture.
5. Divide the salad equally among 4 dinner plates. Distribute the beans, eggs, tomatoes, and olives among the plates, making a

(continued)

cluster of each around the edge of the salad. Garnish the green
beans with a spoonful of onion relish, if desired (see page 197),
and top each serving with 2 anchovies.

4 servings. Per serving: 355 calories, 15 g protein, 13 g carbohydrate, 29 g fat, 5 g fiber

Molly's Piquant Onion Relish

This savory onion relish enlivens grilled meats, especially chicken and pork. It's also a great complement to the Salad Niçoise recipe (page 195).

1 red onion, peeled and thinly sliced
½ cup apple cider vinegar
½ cup water
2 cloves garlic
1 bay leaf
½ teaspoon dried thyme
½ teaspoon dried rosemary
Salt and ground black pepper to taste

1. Soak the onion slices in water for 10 minutes and drain.

2. Put the onion, vinegar, water, garlic, bay leaf, thyme, and rosemary in a saucepan. Bring to a boil, reduce the heat to medium, and cook for 10 minutes, stirring occasionally. Allow to cool. Season with salt and pepper.

8 servings. Per serving: 18 calories, 1 g protein, 5 g carbohydrate, 0 g fat, 1 g fiber

Warm Sweet and Sour Pork Salad

In Thai cooking, salads can be a main course made with all sorts of vegetables and fresh herbs topped with meats and shrimp hot from the grill. Sample this salad made with marinated pork and dressed in a spicy Thai chili sauce, and it's sure to become a favorite dinnertime meal. You don't have to wait to go to a Thai restaurant to enjoy the tangy flavors of Thai cuisine. But a word of warning: Thai cooking typically goes heavy on the fiery chile peppers. Tune the spiciness to your own taste.

Marinade
3 cloves garlic, minced
1" length fresh ginger, peeled and finely chopped
2 tablespoons fish sauce
2 tablespoons soy sauce

Salad
1 pound boneless pork loin
4 sprigs fresh cilantro, stems removed
1 scallion, trimmed
4 cups chopped iceberg lettuce
1 cucumber, peeled
1 mango, peeled
1 avocado, peeled, cut in half, seed removed
1 tablespoon spicy Thai chili sauce, such as Thai Kitchen
    brand, or to taste
¼ cup lime juice
4 small red or green chile peppers, or to taste, seeds
    removed and finely chopped
4 tablespoons roasted peanuts

1. To make the marinade, in a small bowl, mix the garlic, ginger, fish sauce, and soy sauce.
2. To make the salad, cut the pork into thin slices and cut these into strips. If necessary, cut the strips in half so they are

about 1½" to 2" long. Put the pork strips in a shallow dish and add the marinade. Toss to coat the meat, cover, and refrigerate for 1 hour.

3. Meanwhile, finely chop the cilantro and cut the scallion crosswise into ¼" slices. Put in a large bowl, along with the lettuce. Toss to combine.

4. Cut the cucumber crosswise into quarters and cut each quarter vertically into sticks. Slice the mango, then cut the slices crosswise into smaller wedges. Cut each avocado half into slices.

5. Distribute the lettuce mixture equally on 4 dinner plates. Arrange equal amounts of cucumber, mango, and avocado on each bed of lettuce.

6. Mix the chili sauce, lime juice, chile peppers, and ¼ cup water in a small bowl. Set aside.

7. Stir-fry the pork and marinade in a skillet for 3 to 4 minutes, until the pork is no longer pink.

8. Pour the chili sauce and lime juice mixture into the skillet and stir with the meat. Once the sauce is heated, spoon the pork onto each salad. Scatter peanuts over each salad and serve immediately.

4 servings. Per serving: 476 calories, 40 g protein, 22 g carbohydrate, 27 g fat, 7 g fiber

Beet and Pear Salad with Warm Breaded Goat Cheese

The small amount of flour in this recipe bonds the goat cheese as it melts into a creamy morsel that perfectly complements the sweet and tart flavors of the dish. Enjoy this salad topped with toasted walnuts.

> 1 log (6 ounces) goat cheese, chilled
> 3 tablespoons flour
> 1 egg, lightly beaten
> 1 tablespoon milk
> ⅓ cup plain bread crumbs
> Salt and ground black pepper to taste
> ¼ cup walnut oil
> 2 tablespoons sherry wine vinegar
> 1 teaspoon Dijon mustard
> 1 shallot, peeled and finely chopped
> ¼ teaspoon thyme
> 1 large cooked beet or 1 can (15 ounces) sliced beets, drained
> 1 ripe Anjou pear
> 4 cups mâche, mesclun, or other tender, delicately flavored lettuce
> ¼ cup extra virgin olive oil

1. Cut the chilled goat cheese log crosswise into 8 even rounds.

2. Put the flour in a shallow dish. In a small bowl, whisk together the egg and milk. Put the bread crumbs in a separate shallow dish. Season the goat cheese rounds with salt and pepper. Dredge 1 round in flour, shaking off the excess, dip in the egg wash, and then dredge in the bread crumbs, pressing to coat it well. Repeat with the remaining rounds. Return the rounds to the refrigerator to chill for 30 minutes.

3. To prepare the salad dressing, put the walnut oil, vinegar, mustard, shallot, and thyme in a small bowl and whisk to combine.

4. Peel and quarter the beet and cut it into thin wedges. Core the pear and cut it into slim slices. Put the lettuce in a large bowl.

Add the beet and pear and drizzle with the salad dressing. Gently toss. Distribute on 4 salad plates, placing a few of the beet and pear slices on top of the lettuce as a garnish.

5. Put the olive oil in a small pan over medium-high heat. Carefully place the goat cheese rounds into the hot oil, taking care not to crowd the pan. Cook the cheese for 1 to 2 minutes, until the bread crumbs on the underside are lightly browned; turn with a spatula. Cook for an additional 1 to 2 minutes, until the cheese has softened. Transfer 2 slices to each salad plate and serve immediately.

4 servings as starter course, 2 servings as main course. Per starter-course serving: 367 calories, 11 g protein, 22 g carbohydrate, 11 g fat, 3 g fiber

Strawberry Salad

This salad looks as good as it tastes. And between the berries, the greens, and the almonds, it's ridiculously good for you. Make the dressing right before making the salad, since its flavors are most vibrant when fresh.

> 6 tablespoons slivered almonds
> 4½ quarts mixed greens
> Strawberry Vinaigrette (recipe follows)
> 30 strawberries, sliced
> 1½ cups sliced celery from the pale inner heart
> 6 scallions, including the crisp greens, sliced

1. Toast the almonds; just stir them in a dry skillet over medium heat until they're touched with gold.
2. Dump the mixed greens into a huge bowl. Pour on the dressing and toss. Pile the salad on 6 plates or into 6 bowls.
3. Top with the strawberries, celery, scallions, and almonds. Serve immediately.

6 servings. Per serving: 307 calories, 8 g protein, 22 g carbohydrate, 24 g fat, 10 g fiber

Strawberry Vinaigrette

> 20 strawberries
> ½ cup olive oil
> ½ cup balsamic vinegar
> 4 teaspoons Dijon or spicy brown mustard
> 1 teaspoon ground black pepper
> ¼ cup Splenda (or sugar, if you must!)

Assemble the strawberries, oil, vinegar, mustard, pepper, and Splenda in your food processor (with the S blade in place) or blender and run it until the berries are pureed. Best used fresh.

6 servings. Per serving: 182 calories, 1 g protein, 6 g carbohydrate, 18 g fat, 1 g fiber

Coleslaw

Feel free to use bagged coleslaw mix if you don't feel like shredding your own cabbage.

½ head cabbage, shredded
¼ medium red onion, finely chopped
⅓ cup light mayonnaise
⅓ cup plain yogurt
1 teaspoon brown mustard
1 tablespoon apple cider vinegar
1 teaspoon Splenda or sugar
⅛ teaspoon salt or Vege-Sal, or to taste

Throw the cabbage and onion into a big mixing bowl. Stir together the mayonnaise, yogurt, mustard, vinegar, Splenda or sugar, and salt or Vege-Sal. Dump it over the cabbage and toss to coat. Great right away, even better with a few hours of chilling.

5 servings. Per serving: 75 calories, 2 g protein, 7 g carbohydrate, 4 g fat, 2 g fiber

Note: Alternatively, stir up the mayo and yogurt with a good dollop of Balsamic-Mustard Sauce (page 204).

Balsamic-Mustard Sauce

A dollop will add an extra kick to anything from coleslaw to cocktail sauce. The recipe makes quite a lot. And it will keep for a good 6 weeks in an airtight container in the fridge.

½ cup water
1½ teaspoons guar
½ cup + 2 tablespoons balsamic vinegar
1 tablespoon salt
½ cup Splenda
1 egg
¼ cup spicy brown mustard
4 tablespoons butter, in pieces

1. Put the water, guar, vinegar, salt, Splenda, egg, and mustard in your blender and blend until smooth and thick. Pour and scrape into a saucepan over very low heat.

2. Warm the sauce slowly, stirring constantly. When it's hot, whisk in the butter a bit at a time, letting each addition melt and become amalgamated before adding more. When all the butter is blended in, let your sauce cook for another few minutes, then pour into an airtight container and refrigerate.

32 servings (about 1½ tablespoons each). Per serving: 19 calories, trace protein, 1 g carbohydrate, 2 g fat, 0 g fiber

Classic Unpotato Salad

This is a delicious salad, but here's the big picture: We have made at least a dozen different potato salad recipes, substituting cauliflower for the potatoes, and they've all come out great. Please, try your own favorite potato salad recipe with cauliflower!

½ head cauliflower
2 tablespoons wine vinegar
½ teaspoon salt
½ teaspoon ground black pepper
3 hard-cooked eggs, peeled and chopped
1 large rib celery, finely chopped
¼ cup finely chopped bread-and-butter pickles
5 scallions, including the crisp greens, thinly sliced
2 tablespoons finely chopped parsley
½ cup light or regular mayonnaise
2 tablespoons brown mustard

1. Trim the leaves and the very bottom of the stem off the cauliflower. Cut the rest into ½" chunks. Put the chunks in a microwaveable baking dish with a lid, add a couple of tablespoons of water, cover, and microwave on high for 9 minutes.

2. While the cauliflower is cooking, mix together the vinegar, salt, and pepper in a big mixing bowl.

3. When your microwave beeps, pull out the cauliflower, uncover it immediately to stop the cooking, drain it, and dump it into the mixing bowl. Stir it up with the seasoned vinegar. Add the eggs, celery, pickles, scallions, and parsley.

4. Add the mayo and mustard and mix everything up. It's best if you can chill it for an hour or two.

5 servings. Per serving: 139 calories, 6 g protein, 9 g carbohydrate, 8 g fat, 2 g fiber

Easy Pea Salad

This is a retread of a popular salad from the mid-20th century. Back then it was made with canned peas. I think the thawed, uncooked frozen peas are better—fresher tasting, with no mushy texture—but the original version has its charm too. One can of peas, drained, can be substituted for the thawed frozen ones, if you like.

1½ cups frozen peas, thawed
¼ cup finely chopped red onion
¼ cup shredded Cheddar cheese
¼ cup light mayonnaise
1 teaspoon Splenda or sugar
1 teaspoon spicy brown mustard
Salt to taste

Toss the peas, onion, and cheese into a mixing bowl. In a separate bowl, stir the mayonnaise, Splenda or sugar, mustard, and salt together. Place on the pea mixture and stir it up.

3 servings. Per serving: 147 calories, 6 g protein, 13 g carbohydrate, 7 g fat, 4 g fiber

Middle Eastern/Southwestern Fusion Salad

Salads of cucumber, tomato, and onion, dressed with olive oil and lemon juice, are common in Middle Eastern cuisine. The avocado, cilantro, and cumin are southwestern. The two together are fresh and wonderful! Perfect with grilled steak or chicken on a hot summer night. This salad is best served absolutely fresh, so assemble it right before you're planning to serve it—holding it for even a half hour changes it. It's certainly still tasty but not as wonderful.

¼ cup extra virgin olive oil
2 teaspoons ground cumin
1 lemon
½ large cucumber, sliced
2 medium tomatoes, sliced into thin wedges
1 avocado, quartered, peeled, pitted, and sliced crosswise
⅛ large red onion, sliced paper-thin
¼ cup chopped fresh cilantro
½ teaspoon salt

1. Mix together the oil and cumin and reserve. Squeeze the juice from the lemon into another little dish and set that aside too.

2. Assemble the cucumber, tomatoes, avocado, onion, and cilantro in a nonreactive mixing bowl (such as stainless steel or glass). Pour on the olive oil mixture and toss. Pour on the lemon juice and then sprinkle on the salt, toss again, and serve immediately.

6 servings. Per serving: 151 calories, 1 g protein, 7 g carbohydrate, 14 g fat, 2 g fiber

Vietnamese Cucumber Salad

This one is Vietnamese in inspiration, sweet and tart.

> **1 large cucumber, halved and sliced**
> **1 large shallot, finely chopped**
> **½ jalapeño chile pepper, seeded and finely chopped (wear plastic gloves when handling)**
> **1 tablespoon lime juice**
> **¼ cup rice vinegar**
> **3 tablespoons Splenda or sugar**
> **½ teaspoon salt**
> **3 tablespoons finely chopped fresh cilantro**

1. In a nonreactive mixing bowl (such as stainless steel or glass), combine the cucumber with the shallot and jalapeño pepper.

2. Combine the lime juice, vinegar, Splenda or sugar, and salt and pour over the salad. Stir. Add the cilantro and stir again. You can serve this right away, but 15 to 20 minutes of chilling time lets the flavors blend. Best eaten the same day, though.

4 servings. Per serving: 20 calories, 1 g protein, 5 g carbohydrate, trace fat, 1 g fiber

Fruit Salad with Poppy Seed Dressing

Here's a salad that makes the most of summer's bounty.

> 2 nectarines (you could use peaches, but you'd need to
>   peel them)
> 10 strawberries
> 1 cup blueberries
> 4 teaspoons Splenda or sugar
> 4 teaspoons lemon juice
> 2 tablespoons oil
> 2 pinches mustard powder
> ½ teaspoon poppy seeds
> ⅛ teaspoon salt

1. Halve the nectarines and remove the pits, then finely chop them—you don't have to bother to peel them first. Put them in a pretty glass bowl.

2. Halve the strawberries lengthwise, then slice and add to the nectarines. Throw in the blueberries.

3. Now whisk together the Splenda or sugar, lemon juice, oil, mustard powder, poppy seeds, and salt and pour over the fruit. Toss to coat and stash in the fridge for an hour or so before serving.

4 servings. Per serving: 128 calories, 1 g protein, 16 g carbohydrate, 8 g fat, 3 g fiber

Tomatoes Stuffed with Curried Tuna Salad

This trick of stuffing tomato "flowers" makes any tuna, chicken, egg, or ham salad special (and more nutritious). But when you spark that tuna salad with curry, ginger, currants, and cashews, it becomes really amazing.

> 1 can (6 ounces) chunk light tuna packed in water
> 1 rib celery, finely chopped
> 3 scallions, including the crisp greens, sliced
> 1 tablespoon dried currants
> 3 tablespoons light mayonnaise
> 1½ teaspoons curry powder
> ½ teaspoon grated fresh ginger
> 2 medium tomatoes
> 2 lettuce leaves for serving
> 2 tablespoons chopped roasted, salted cashews

1. Drain the tuna and dump it into a mixing bowl. Add the celery, scallions, and currants.

2. Stir together the mayonnaise, curry powder, and ginger. Now add to the tuna and mix to combine.

3. Cut the cores out of the tomatoes. Cut each vertically into 8 wedges, leaving the skin intact at the bottom. Open up each tomato into a "flower."

4. Line 2 serving plates with pretty lettuce leaves and place a tomato on each.

5. At the last minute, stir the cashews into the tuna salad. Then divide the mixture between the tomatoes and serve.

2 servings. Per serving: 255 calories, 25 g protein, 17 g carbohydrate, 10 g fat, 3 g fiber

Colorful Dill Egg Salad

A great recipe to have on hand after Easter! We like to wrap this salad in lettuce leaves, but it would be truly gorgeous stuffed into a tomato.

6 hard-cooked eggs, peeled and chopped
2 large ribs celery, finely chopped
½ red bell pepper, finely chopped
6 scallions, including the crisp greens, sliced
¼ cup ranch dressing
¼ cup light mayonnaise
½ teaspoon lemon pepper
1 teaspoon dried dill

1. Put the chopped eggs into a mixing bowl. Add the celery, bell pepper, and scallions.

2. Mix together the ranch dressing, mayonnaise, lemon pepper, and dill and pour it over the salad. Stir it up and serve.

3 servings. Per serving: 325 calories, 15 g protein, 9 g carbohydrate, 25 g fat, 2 g fiber

Chicken–Smoked Gouda Salad

A great flavor combination. Feel free to use bagged mixed greens instead of the romaine and red leaf.

> ½ pound boneless, skinless chicken breast
> Salt and ground black pepper to taste
> 1 teaspoon olive oil
> 2 slices bacon
> 4 cups torn romaine lettuce
> 4 cups torn red leaf lettuce
> ¼ cup shredded smoked Gouda cheese
> ¼ cup very thinly sliced red onion
> Apricot-Mustard Dressing (opposite)

1. Put the chicken in a resealable plastic bag and use the nearest heavy, blunt object to pound it out to an even ½" thickness. Salt and pepper it lightly, then start cooking it in the oil. You'll want to give it 4 minutes per side and cook until golden and cooked through but not dried out. (Or you could cook it on your electric tabletop grill.)

2. Cook the bacon. Meanwhile, put the greens, Gouda, and onion in a big salad bowl. Pour on the dressing and toss until every leaf is coated. Pile the salad on 2 plates.

3. When your chicken is done, slice or cube it and top the salads with it. Crumble a slice of bacon over each and serve.

2 servings. Per serving: 375 calories, 34 g protein, 12 g carbohydrate, 21 g fat, 4 g fiber

Apricot-Mustard Dressing

We're putting this dressing by itself because we want you to think of it not just as a salad dressing but also when you need a dipping sauce for chicken, pork, or seafood.

> **1 tablespoon low-sugar apricot preserves**
> **1 tablespoon apple cider vinegar**
> **1 tablespoon olive oil**
> **1 tablespoon light mayonnaise**
> **1 teaspoon Dijon or spicy brown mustard**
> **1 teaspoon Splenda or sugar**
> **Scant ⅛ teaspoon ground black pepper**
> **Pinch of salt or Vege-Sal**

Mix together the preserves, vinegar, oil, mayonnaise, mustard, Splenda or sugar, pepper, and salt or Vege-Sal.

2 to 3 servings of salad, the whole batch has 185 calories, trace protein, 8 g carbohydrate, 17 g fat, trace fiber

Chicken Slaw with Honey-Mustard Dressing

Throw in an extra piece or two when you're roasting chicken, buy a sack of shredded coleslaw, and this is a snap. Feel free to make this with leftover turkey too.

1 cup finely chopped cooked chicken
2 cups shredded cabbage
2 scallions, including the crisp greens, thinly sliced
½ teaspoon butter
2 tablespoons slivered almonds
3 tablespoons light mayonnaise (or regular, if you prefer)
2 teaspoons spicy brown or Dijon mustard
2 teaspoons honey or Splenda
1 teaspoon balsamic vinegar
Salt and ground black pepper to taste

1. In a mixing bowl, combine the chicken, cabbage, and scallions.

2. Melt the butter in a skillet and stir over medium heat and toast the almonds until they're golden. Throw them in the mixing bowl too.

3. In a small dish, stir together the mayonnaise, mustard, honey or Splenda, and vinegar. Pour over the salad and toss to coat. Add salt and pepper to taste and serve.

2 servings. Per serving: 275 calories, 25 g protein, 14 g carbohydrate, 13 g fat, 3 g fiber

Grilled Chicken Salad with Spinach and Apples

A few simple ingredients add up to a salad that's truly delicious—and overwhelmingly nutritious.

> ½ **pound boneless, skinless chicken breast**
> **Salt and ground black pepper to taste**
> **3 tablespoons olive oil**
> **3 tablespoons apple cider vinegar**
> **2 teaspoons Splenda or sugar**
> **1 small clove garlic, crushed**
> **6 cups bagged baby spinach**
> **1 small apple, cored and finely chopped**
> **2 scallions, including the crisp greens, sliced**
> ¼ **cup shredded Romano or Parmesan cheese**

1. Cut the chicken into two 4-ounce portions. You can place it in a resealable plastic bag and pound it lightly to an even thickness, about ½", or you can skip this if you want. Either way, salt and pepper both sides, then either throw the chicken into a hot skillet coated with a little cooking spray (or olive oil) or toss it onto your electric tabletop grill. You'll want to cook it for 4 to 5 minutes per side, until golden and cooked through but not dried out.

2. Put the oil, vinegar, Splenda or sugar, and garlic into a bowl and whisk together well.

3. Dump the spinach into a salad bowl and pour on the dressing. Toss well, then pile the spinach onto 2 plates.

4. Top each serving with half the apple and half the scallions. When your chicken is done, slice or cube it. Top each salad with half the chicken. Scatter 2 tablespoons of the cheese over each salad and serve.

2 servings. Per serving: 440 calories, 33 g protein, 18 g carbohydrate, 28 g fat, 5 g fiber

Oriental Chicken Salad

This is the sort of thing that you'd pay $12.95 for in a restaurant. Yet despite the intimidating list of ingredients, it's quite simple.

½ pound boneless, skinless chicken breast
Salt and ground black pepper to taste
1 teaspoon olive oil
1 teaspoon butter
2 tablespoons sliced almonds
3 tablespoons Splenda or sugar
2 tablespoons rice wine vinegar
¼ cup light or regular mayonnaise
1 teaspoon spicy brown or Dijon mustard
⅛ teaspoon dark sesame oil
⅛ teaspoon chili garlic paste
⅛ teaspoon soy sauce
3 cups chopped romaine lettuce
1 cup shredded red cabbage
1 cup shredded napa cabbage
1 cup fresh mung bean sprouts
½ carrot, shredded
2 scallions, including the crisp greens, sliced

1. Put the chicken breast in a resealable plastic bag and use any handy heavy object to pound it to an even ½" thickness. Salt and pepper both sides lightly. Add the oil to a skillet over medium-high heat and add the chicken breast. You want to give it 4 to 5 minutes per side, until it's golden and done through but not dried out. (Alternatively, you can use your electric tabletop grill to do this step.)

2. In your smallest skillet, melt the butter over medium-low heat and add the sliced almonds.

3. While the chicken and almonds are cooking, make your dressing. Measure the Splenda or sugar, vinegar, mayonnaise, mustard, sesame oil, chili garlic paste, and soy sauce into a small bowl and whisk until smooth. Now stir your almonds—you don't want to burn them; just brown them a little.

4. Assemble the lettuce, red cabbage, napa cabbage, bean sprouts, carrot, and scallions in a big salad bowl. Pour on the dressing and toss vigorously until everything is coated evenly. Pile the salad on 2 plates.

5. Throw the cooked chicken onto your chopping board, slice or cube it, and divide it between the 2 salads. Top each with a tablespoon of almonds and serve.

2 servings. Per serving: 368 calories, 32 g protein, 19 g carbohydrate, 19 g fat, 5 g fiber

Walnut-Chicken Salad

This was originally a couscous salad, but the cauliflower is terrific. The recipe looks complicated, but only takes about 10 minutes to put together.

½ head cauliflower
1 tablespoon finely chopped red onion
1 clove garlic, crushed
1½ tablespoons rice wine vinegar
2 tablespoons olive oil
1 teaspoon Splenda or sugar
½ teaspoon grated fresh ginger
½ teaspoon lemon juice
1 teaspoon soy sauce
½ pound boneless, skinless chicken breast
Salt and ground black pepper to taste
2 teaspoons butter, divided
½ cup shredded carrot
1 bunch scallions, including the crisp greens, sliced
¼ cup chopped walnuts
6 cups fresh baby spinach

1. Trim the leaves and the very bottom of the stem off the cauliflower and break it into chunks. Run it through the shredding disk of your food processor. Dump the resulting "rice" into a microwaveable baking dish with a lid, add a tablespoon or two of water, cover, and microwave on high for 6 minutes.

2. Now make your dressing: Put the onion and garlic in a small bowl. Add the vinegar, olive oil, Splenda or sugar, ginger, lemon juice, and soy sauce. Whisk everything together.

3. Put your chicken breast in a resealable plastic bag and use a heavy, blunt object to pound it out to a ½" thickness all over. Salt and pepper lightly on both sides. Spray a medium skillet with cooking spray, put it over medium heat, and add 1 teaspoon of the butter. When the skillet's hot, throw in your chicken breast—it'll take 4 to 5 minutes per side. Meanwhile, throw the carrot and scallions into a big salad bowl.

4. Pull out the cauliflower and uncover it right away to stop the cooking.

5. When the chicken is done, throw it on your chopping board. Melt the other teaspoon of butter and toss the walnuts into the skillet. Stir them in the butter until they smell toasty, then remove from the heat.

6. Drain your cauliflower "rice" and dump it in the salad bowl. Give your dressing another stir, pour it over the cauliflower mixture, and toss everything together. Add a little salt and pepper if you think it needs it. Now stir in the walnuts.

7. Pile the baby spinach on 2 plates. Spoon the cauliflower mixture on top. Slice your chicken breast and divide the chicken between the 2 servings.

2 servings. Per serving: 459 calories, 35 g protein, 18 g carbohydrate, 30 g fat, 8 g fiber

Ham and Pineapple Slaw

Once you bake a ham, you spend the next week figuring out how to use it up. This recipe makes that same old ham fresh again in a way starchy sandwiches and casseroles never could.

3 cups shredded napa cabbage
½ cup shredded red cabbage
½ cup finely chopped pineapple
2 scallions, including the crisp greens, sliced
6 ounces cooked ham, cut into ½" cubes
2 tablespoons rice vinegar
2 tablespoons light or regular mayonnaise
1 tablespoon spicy brown mustard
1 tablespoon Splenda
½ teaspoon soy sauce
⅛ teaspoon chili garlic paste
¼ clove garlic, crushed
1 tablespoon sesame seeds

1. Throw the napa cabbage, red cabbage, pineapple, scallions, and ham into a big salad bowl or mixing bowl. In a small dish, whisk together the vinegar, mayonnaise, mustard, Splenda, soy sauce, chili garlic paste, and garlic.

2. Put the sesame seeds in a small, dry skillet and shake them over medium heat for a few minutes, until they smell toasty. (If you're using hulled sesame seeds—the only kind you'll find at your grocery store—they may well pop and jump a bit in the skillet, and they'll turn golden. If you use unhulled sesame seeds from the health food store—our choice, for the higher mineral content—they won't be so dramatic. Just give them a few minutes and they'll be fine.)

3. Now pour the dressing over the salad and toss until everything's coated. Throw in the sesame seeds, toss again, and serve.

2 servings. Per serving: 284 calories, 19 g protein, 20 g carbohydrate, 15 g fat, 4 g fiber

Note: Buy precut chunks of fresh pineapple in the produce department and just chop them up further, to about ¼"-thick pieces.

18

Side Dishes

Dropping potatoes, rice, and noodles from your diet can be disorienting. Sure, steak, chicken, chops, and the like are friendly and familiar. But what goes on that third of the plate where the starch used to be?

Vegetables! But not just plain buttered vegetables (although they're fine). Interesting vegetables. Heck, exciting vegetables, both hot and cold. It's time to broaden your repertoire of vegetable dishes and salads.

Vegetables to the Rescue

If you move beyond simply steaming vegetables or cooking them in the microwave, you'll find they can be anything but boring. Try some of the great sides in this list in addition to the following recipes.

- **Feta green beans:** Steam green beans until they're still slightly crunchy. Serve at room temperature and sprinkle with feta cheese, fresh mint, and pine nuts.
- **Parmesan asparagus:** Roast asparagus in the oven at high heat in balsamic vinegar and olive oil until crispy, and then sprinkle with Parmesan cheese.

- **Broccoli and almonds:** Cook broccoli with butter, lemon juice, and toasted almond slices, stirring frequently.
- **Cauliflower au gratin:** Steam cauliflower (or another vegetable), combine it with a white sauce, top it with cheese, and bake until golden brown.
- **Mushroom medley:** Cook a variety of mushrooms in butter.
- **Fresh artichokes:** Steam artichokes and serve them with melted butter or your favorite dipping sauce.
- **Portobello mushrooms:** Roast or grill the mushrooms and sprinkle them with fresh herbs and goat cheese.
- **Scalloped summer squash:** Cube and steam squash and then bake with cooked onions, garlic, and bell pepper topped with Parmesan cheese.
- **Ricotta tomatoes:** Stuff tomato halves with spinach and ricotta cheese and bake until the filling begins to bubble.

Just as there are thousands of recipes for potatoes or rice, these basic recipes lend themselves to endless variations. And not only do they have a low glycemic load and far more nutrients than your old starchy favorites, but they cook faster too!

Fauxtatoes

This first foundation recipe is an old standard in the low-carb community. It's a stand-in for mashed potatoes. Even if you're sure you don't like cauliflower, try it. More than once, we've served a guest "fauxtatoes" topped with a flavorful gravy, only to have him or her yum down five or six mouthfuls before looking up, puzzled, to say, "Wait. Those aren't mashed potatoes. What are they?" They never guess it's cauliflower. These are remarkably good just as they are and fabulous with gravy. Try melting in a little cream cheese if you want a richer texture.

> ½ head cauliflower
> 2 tablespoons butter, or to taste
> Salt and ground black pepper to taste

1. Trim the leaves and the very bottom of the stem off your cauliflower and whack the rest into chunks. Put them in a microwaveable baking dish with a lid, add a few tablespoons of water, and cover. Microwave on high for 10 to 12 minutes, or until tender.

2. When the cauliflower is cooked, drain it well. Use your blender, food processor, or stick blender to puree the cauliflower. Melt in the butter, add salt and pepper to taste, and serve.

3 servings. Per serving: 92 calories, 2 g protein, 5 g carbohydrate, 8 g fat, 2 g fiber

Cauliflower-Potato Mash

Want something a little more potato-y? The addition of just a little potato makes your pureed cauliflower a truly convincing mashed potato clone—with a vastly lower glycemic load and fewer calories and more vitamins to boot!

½ head cauliflower
1 medium potato
2 tablespoons butter
Salt and ground black pepper to taste

1. Trim the leaves and the very bottom of the stem off the cauliflower and whack it into chunks. Scrub or peel the potato and whack it into chunks. Put both in a microwaveable baking dish with a lid. Add a tablespoon or two of water, cover, and microwave on high for 12 to 15 minutes, or until both are good and tender.

2. Drain the veggies. Now use your blender, stick blender, or food processor to puree them together. Stir in the butter and salt and pepper to taste, and serve.

4 servings. Per serving: 97 calories, 2 g protein, 10 g carbohydrate, 6 g fat, 2 g fiber

Note: Whether you make Fauxtatoes or Cauliflower-Potato Mash, feel free to play with the recipe. Anything you'd put in mashed potatoes—garlic, cheese, horseradish, you name it—is good in these purees.

Cauliflower "Rice"

Here is the second foundation recipe. Credit where credit is due: We found this idea in Fran McCullough's wonderful book *The Low-Carb Cookbook*. I've used it literally hundreds of ways since, in everything from fried "rice" to "rice" salads. This is the basic version. Butter, salt, and pepper it, if you like, or use it as a bed for a stir-fry.

½ head cauliflower

1. Trim the leaves and the very bottom of the stem from the cauliflower. Whack the rest into pieces that'll fit into the feed tube of your food processor.
2. Fit your food processor with its shredding disk. Now run the cauliflower through the shredding blade. Put the resulting cauliflower "rice" in a microwaveable baking dish with a lid. Add a couple of tablespoons of water and microwave on high for just 6 to 7 minutes. Uncover as soon as the microwave oven beeps to avoid overcooking.

3 servings. Per serving: 24 calories, 2 g protein, 5 g carbohydrate, trace fat, 2 g fiber

Rice-a-Phony

Here's a simple example of how to use cauliflower "rice." There's a basic principle here that you should pay attention to: the use of bouillon concentrate to flavor the "rice." Real rice is often cooked in broth, but this won't do for cauliflower rice, since it doesn't absorb liquid. Stirring in bouillon concentrate gives you the flavor of broth without the water.

½ head cauliflower
2 teaspoons butter
¼ cup slivered almonds
1 bunch scallions, including the crisp greens, sliced
¼ cup chopped parsley
2 teaspoons chicken bouillon concentrate

1. Make Cauliflower "Rice" (page 225). Trim your cauliflower, whack it into chunks, run it through the shredding disk of your food processor, and microwave the resulting cauliflower "rice" on high for 6 minutes.

2. Meanwhile, put your big, heavy skillet over medium heat, add the butter, and start cooking the almonds in it, stirring frequently.

3. Once the almonds are golden, drain the cauliflower and dump it into the skillet with the almonds. Stir in the scallions, parsley, and bouillon concentrate, mixing until the bouillon concentrate is dissolved and everything is well distributed.

3 servings. Per serving: 124 calories, 5 g protein, 8 g carbohydrate, 9 g fat, 3 g fiber

Note: For a nice variation, try pine nuts in place of the almonds.

Pecan "Rice"

With a good broiled steak and a glass of red wine, this makes for a glorious dinner. For that matter, if you have leftover steak or roast beef in the house, you could finely chop it and stir it into this rice dish for a skillet supper.

½ head cauliflower
¼ cup chopped pecans
1 bunch scallions
1 tablespoon butter
1 tablespoon olive oil
½ cup frozen peas
⅓ cup cooked wild rice
2 teaspoons beef bouillon concentrate
¼ cup dry white wine
Hot-pepper sauce to taste (start with a few dashes)
Salt and ground black pepper to taste
¼ cup chopped parsley

1. Trim the leaves and the very bottom of the stem from the cauliflower. Whack the cauliflower into chunks and run it through the shredding disk of your food processor.

2. Dump the resulting "rice" into a microwaveable baking dish with a lid, add a tablespoon or two of water, cover, and microwave on high for 6 minutes.

3. Meanwhile, spread the pecans in a shallow baking pan and place them in a 350°F oven for 10 minutes to toast. Set the timer, or you'll forget them, sure as you're born. (If you like, buy toasted salted pecans and just chop them.)

4. Slice the scallions, including the crisp part of the greens, and set them aside.

5. Give your biggest skillet a shot of cooking spray and put it over medium-low heat. Add the butter and oil.

6. When the microwave oven beeps, pull out the cauliflower and uncover it to stop the cooking. Put the peas in a small dish, add a tablespoon of water, cover, and microwave for just 90 seconds to 2 minutes on high.

(continued)

7. Drain the cauliflower and dump it into the skillet. Add the wild rice, bouillon concentrate, and wine and stir everything really well. Now give it a shot of the hot-pepper sauce and taste. Add more if it needs it. Let the whole thing cook together for 5 minutes to let the wine cook down a bit.

8. Meanwhile, drain the peas and throw them in, then salt and pepper the whole thing. Right before serving, stir in the parsley, the scallions, and those toasted pecans, and serve.

5 servings. Per serving: 131 calories, 3 g protein, 9 g carbohydrate, 9 g fat, 3 g fiber

Note: Look for teeny boxes of wild rice with the other rice in your grocery store. Don't buy "wild and long-grain rice blend." All the grains should be dark brown. Cook according to package directions and stash it in an airtight container in your freezer. Then you'll have wild rice on hand whenever you want it!

Parmesan Broccoli

You could use fresh broccoli, but you'd have to cut it up and blanch it—cook it in boiling water for just a few minutes—then drain it, before you could stir-fry it. After blanching, it would be very much like thawed frozen broccoli. So why work that hard?

    2 tablespoons olive oil
    1 pound frozen broccoli "cuts," thawed
    1 clove garlic, crushed
    1 teaspoon red-pepper flakes
    3 tablespoons grated Parmesan cheese
    ¼ teaspoon salt

1. Put your big, heavy skillet over high heat and add the oil. When it's hot, add the broccoli. Stir-fry it until it's tender-crisp, with a few brown spots.

2. Stir in the garlic and red-pepper flakes and stir-fry for another minute or two.

3. Stir in the Parmesan and salt, and serve.

3 servings. Per serving: 143 calories, 6 g protein, 8 g carbohydrate, 11 g fat, 5 g fiber

Broccoli with Cashews

This fast and delicious Asian-style broccoli is far easier than it tastes.

  1 pound frozen broccoli
  2 tablespoons butter
  1½ teaspoons Sucanat
  2 tablespoons soy sauce
  1½ teaspoons rice vinegar
  1 clove garlic, minced
  ⅛ teaspoon chili garlic paste
  ¼ cup roasted salted cashews

1. Microwave the broccoli on high until tender-crisp.

2. While the broccoli is cooking, melt the butter in a small saucepan and whisk in the Sucanat, soy sauce, vinegar, garlic, and chili garlic paste. Chop the cashews.

3. When your broccoli is tender-crisp and brilliant green, drain it and toss with your sauce. Add the cashews and toss again, then serve.

3 servings. Per serving: 174 calories, 5 g protein, 12 g carbohydrate, 13 g fat, 4 g fiber

Stir-Fried Snow Peas
with Water Chestnuts and Cashews

If you like Chinese food, you'll love this.

3 cups fresh snow pea pods
2 tablespoons peanut oil
2 cloves garlic, minced
1 tablespoon grated fresh ginger
1 can (8 ounces) sliced water chestnuts, drained
¼ teaspoon chili garlic paste
1½ teaspoons soy sauce
¼ cup roasted cashews, chopped

1. Pinch the ends off the snow peas and pull the strings off the sides.

2. Put a big skillet or wok over high heat. When it's hot, add the oil, then the snow peas, garlic, and ginger. Stir-fry until the snow peas are just barely tender-crisp.

3. Stir in the water chestnuts, chili garlic paste, and soy sauce and continue stir-frying until the water chestnuts are heated through. Stir in the cashews and serve.

3 servings. Per serving: 212 calories, 4 g protein, 19 g carbohydrate, 14 g fat, 4 g fiber

Chipotle Mushrooms

You think simple cooked mushrooms are good on a steak or in an omelet? Try these. Unreal!

2 tablespoons olive oil
8 ounces sliced mushrooms
½ medium onion, chopped
2 cloves garlic, minced
1 chipotle chile pepper canned in adobo, finely chopped
2 tablespoons finely chopped fresh cilantro
Salt and ground black pepper to taste

1. Put your big, heavy skillet over medium heat and add the oil. When it's hot, throw in the mushrooms, onion, garlic, and chipotle pepper. Cook, stirring often, for 8 to 9 minutes, until the mushrooms and onion are soft.

2. Stir in the cilantro and salt and pepper, and serve.

3 servings. Per serving: 109 calories, 2 g protein, 6 g carbohydrate, 9 g fat, 2 g fiber

Blue Cheese Mushrooms

Fantastic—and fantastically easy! Wonderful over a rib-eye steak or chicken breast, in an omelet, or on the side with almost anything.

> 2 teaspoons olive oil
> 2 teaspoons butter
> 4 ounces mushrooms (about 8), sliced
> 1 medium onion, sliced
> 2 cloves garlic, crushed
> 2 tablespoons crumbled blue cheese
> Seasoned salt to taste
> Ground black pepper to taste
> 4 dashes hot-pepper sauce
> ¼ cup chopped parsley

1. In a big skillet over medium heat, combine the oil and butter, swirling them together as the butter melts. Throw in the mushrooms, onion, and garlic.

2. Cook, stirring frequently, until the onion is starting to brown and the mushrooms have softened and changed color. Add the blue cheese and stir until it's mostly melted in. Stir in the salt, pepper, hot-pepper sauce, and parsley and serve.

2 servings. Per serving: 150 calories, 4 g protein, 10 g carbohydrate, 11 g fat, 2 g fiber

Green Beans and Portobellos Vinaigrette

Quick, easy, and elegant.

> 2 tablespoons olive oil
> 1¾ pounds frozen green beans, thawed
> 1 cup chopped portobello mushroom caps
> 1 clove garlic, crushed
> 3 tablespoons sherry vinegar
> Salt and ground black pepper to taste

1. Put your big, heavy skillet over medium-high heat and add the oil. Slosh it around to cover the bottom of the skillet.

2. Add the green beans and mushrooms. Cook, stirring frequently, until the beans are tender-crisp—8 to 10 minutes.

3. Stir in the garlic and vinegar and let the whole thing cook for another 3 to 5 minutes. Add salt and pepper and serve.

6 servings. Per serving: 88 calories, 3 g protein, 11 g carbohydrate, 5 g fat, 4 g fiber

Green Beans with Pine Nuts

A great change from the traditional almonds.

>   **2 pounds fresh or frozen green beans**
>   **1 clove garlic**
>   **2 tablespoons olive oil**
>   **¼ cup pine nuts**
>   **1 tablespoon butter**

1. If you're using fresh beans, trim the ends and cut the beans into 2" lengths. If using frozen, simply start cooking them. Either way, put your beans in a microwaveable baking dish with a lid. Add a couple of tablespoons of water, cover, and microwave on high until just done through but still slightly crisp—10 to 12 minutes. Stir halfway through that time.

2. While the beans are steaming, crush the garlic and put it in a small cup. Pour the oil over it and let it sit.

3. Put the pine nuts in a dry skillet and stir over medium-low heat until they're touched with gold.

4. When the beans are done, drain them well. Toss with the garlic and oil and butter until the butter is melted. Stir in the pine nuts and serve.

8 servings. Per serving: 98 calories, 3 g protein, 8 g carbohydrate, 7 g fat, 4 g fiber

Orange-Hazelnut Green Beans

Perfect for a holiday—or a weeknight, for that matter.

> **4 cups frozen crosscut green beans**
> **4 teaspoons butter**
> **¼ cup chopped hazelnuts**
> **1 teaspoon grated orange peel**
> **6 tablespoons orange juice**
> **1 teaspoon rice vinegar or white wine vinegar**

1. Start steaming the beans, microwaving them on high for 7 to 8 minutes; using a stovetop steamer is fine too.

2. Meanwhile, melt the butter over medium heat in a small, heavy skillet. Add the hazelnuts and cook, stirring frequently, until they're golden.

3. Stir in the orange peel, orange juice, and vinegar. Simmer for just a minute or two, to cook down the sauce and intensify the flavor.

4. When your beans are tender but still bright green, toss with the sauce and serve.

4 servings. Per serving: 131 calories, 3 g protein, 13 g carbohydrate, 9 g fat, 4 g fiber

Grilled Asparagus

You'll be surprised at how good this is!

> **1 pound fresh asparagus**
> **2 tablespoons olive oil**
> **Salt and ground black pepper to taste**

1. Preheat your grill or electric tabletop grill.

2. Snap the ends off the asparagus where the spears break naturally. Put them in a flat pan and toss them with the oil until they're coated. Sprinkle with salt and pepper.

3. Lay the spears across the hot grill, close the lid, and cook for 4 to 5 minutes—until there are brown grill marks on the asparagus—and serve.

3 servings. Per serving: 114 calories, 3 g protein, 7 g carbohydrate, 9 g fat, 3 g fiber

Italian Asparagus

Unusual and wonderful.

>   **2 pounds asparagus**
>   **3 tablespoons olive oil**
>   **2 cloves garlic, crushed**
>   **¼ cup capers, finely chopped**
>   **2 hard-cooked eggs, peeled and grated on the large holes**
>   **of your box grater**
>   **¼ cup grated Romano cheese**

1. Snap the ends off the asparagus where the spears break naturally. Cut into 1" lengths.

2. Give your biggest skillet a squirt of cooking spray (unless it's nonstick; then skip it) and put over medium-high heat. Add the oil. When the oil is hot, add the asparagus and stir-fry until it's brilliant green and tender-crisp.

3. Add the garlic and stir-fry for another minute or so, then stir in the capers.

4. Pile the asparagus into bowls or onto plates. Top each serving with grated egg and cheese and serve.

4 servings. Per serving: 186 calories, 8 g protein, 6 g carbohydrate, 15 g fat, 3 g fiber

Orange-Glazed Carrots

Good ol' carrots. They're cheap year-round and always available. They're usually part of the steamed vegetables that come on the side at restaurants. We love them, but they can get a little . . . boring. Well, forget that! These carrots are outstanding—so sweet and tasty they're almost a dessert.

> **1 pound carrots**
> **¼ cup chopped pecans**
> **1 orange**
> **1 tablespoon butter**
> **1 tablespoon dark rum**
> **4 teaspoons Splenda and ½ teaspoon blackstrap molasses,**
> **or 4 teaspoons Sucanat**

1. Preheat the oven to 350°F.

2. Peel the carrots and cut them into strips or slices, whatever you prefer—we like thin strips. Put them in a microwaveable baking dish with a lid, add a couple of tablespoons of water, cover, and microwave on high for 10 minutes.

3. Spread the pecans in a roasting pan and place them in the oven. Set the timer for 10 minutes.

4. Grate the orange's peel and squeeze the juice into a saucepan big enough to hold your carrots. Put on the stove over medium-low heat and add the butter, rum, and either Splenda and molasses or Sucanat. Stir together until this sauce is cooked down a little and getting syrupy.

5. Pull carrots out of the microwave oven, drain them, and dump them into the saucepan. Stir until the carrots are coated with the sauce.

6. Remove the pecans from the oven, stir them into the carrots, and serve.

4 servings. Per serving: 146 calories, 2 g protein, 16 g carbohydrate, 8 g fat, 4 g fiber

Southern Leafy Greens and Bacon

Dark leafy greens like kale have a slightly bitter, earthy flavor that holds its own with robust meat entrées. The crispy bacon, onion, garlic, currants, and apple cider vinegar add savory, sweet, and tart notes, turning greens into a highly entertaining dish.

> ½ teaspoon salt
> 1½ pounds kale, stems removed, thoroughly washed
>   and coarsely chopped
> 2 slices bacon, cut crosswise into strips
> 1 tablespoon extra virgin olive oil
> 1 medium onion, finely chopped
> 1 clove garlic, minced
> 2 tablespoons currants
> Apple cider vinegar, about 2 teaspoons

1. Fill a large pot with water and bring to a boil. Put the salt and then the kale into the pot and cook, stirring, for 2 minutes, or until the greens wilt. Cover the pot and cook until the kale is tender, about 7 minutes.

2. Meanwhile, fry the bacon in a large skillet over medium heat until crisp, about 5 minutes. Cover a plate with paper towels and place the bacon on this to absorb the excess fat.

3. When the kale is tender, pour it into a colander. Rinse the pot with cold water so that it quickly cools and refill with cold water. Return the kale to the pot to stop the greens from cooking further. Lift the kale out of the pot in handfuls, squeezing it until almost dry, and then collect the kale in a bowl. Set aside.

4. Discard the bacon fat in the skillet and add the oil. Add the onion and cook over medium heat, stirring frequently, until soft, about 3 minutes. Add the garlic and cook for 30 seconds.

5. Add the kale, bacon, and currants. Cover the skillet and reheat the greens, cooking for about 2 minutes. If liquid accumulates, cook uncovered for an additional minute. Sprinkle with the vinegar, stir once, and serve immediately.

4 servings. Per serving: 114 calories, 4 g protein, 15 g carbohydrate, 6 g fat, 4 g fiber

Asian Asparagus Vinaigrette

To spark the flavor of hot vegetables, treat them to a vinegar-and-oil dressing. This simple recipe takes well to variation. You can use broccoli or green beans instead of asparagus. You can also add some garlic, a dash of sesame oil, or a tablespoon of bottled hoisin sauce—a sweet and spicy condiment used in Chinese cooking and available in many supermarkets.

> **1 pound asparagus, tough ends snapped off**
> **1 tablespoon grated fresh ginger**
> **2 tablespoons seasoned rice wine vinegar**
> **1 tablespoon soy sauce**
> **1 tablespoon unrefined safflower oil**

1. Fit a large pot with a steamer basket and fill it with enough water to nearly reach the bottom of the basket. Bring the water to a boil. Add the asparagus and cover with a tight-fitting lid. Cook over medium-high heat for about 5 minutes, or until the stalks compress slightly when squeezed and the asparagus bends slightly when picked up.

2. Meanwhile, in a small bowl, whisk together the ginger, vinegar, soy sauce, and oil.

3. When the asparagus is done, transfer it to a platter and drizzle with the dressing. Serve with steamed fish, steak, and Asian dishes.

4 servings. Per serving: 72 calories, 3 g protein, 9 g carbohydrate, 4 g fat, 2 g fiber

Braised Leeks

Leeks—the uptown version of onions—have a subtle, sweet flavor that makes them an elegant side dish and a lovely complement to soups and stews. Yet they are not a staple in American kitchens, in part because they are pricier than ordinary onions and because prepping these large, seemingly ungainly stalks is unfamiliar territory. So here's a chance to get to know leeks and enjoy them forevermore. This unadorned recipe features the delicate flavor of these special onions.

> **4 thick leeks or 6 medium leeks**
> **3 tablespoons extra virgin olive oil**
> **½ cup vegetable stock or water**
> **2 sprigs parsley**
> **Salt and ground black pepper to taste**
> **1 tablespoon freshly squeezed lemon juice**

1. To trim the leeks, remove any leaves that are withered or yellowed. Cut off the root end and the tough upper portion of the green tops, leaving only a few inches of darker green above the pale green stalk.

2. Leeks often contain a lot of sand. To wash, cut the length of each leek, beginning about 1" from the root end and making a slit down the center of each stalk. With your fingertips, fan out the leaves somewhat and rinse in a bowl or under cold running water. When the leeks are thoroughly cleaned, cut them into 4" lengths.

3. Put the leeks in a saucepan or shallow baking dish, arranging them so they lie flat and straight. Add the oil and stock or water—enough to cover the leeks. Add the parsley and season with salt and pepper. Cover the pan and cook, turning occasionally, until the leeks are very tender and can be easily pierced with a fork, 15 to 25 minutes, depending on the freshness and thickness of the leeks.

4. When the leeks are tender, uncover the pan, raise the heat, and boil away all the liquid. In the process, the leeks will begin to brown lightly. Sprinkle with the lemon juice.

4 servings. Per serving: 126 calories, 1 g protein, 9 g carbohydrate, 10 g fat, 1 g fiber

Cheese-Stuffed Peppers Two Ways

This colorful dish is a great accompaniment to grilled foods and is especially good when fresh peppers and tomatoes are in season.

3 bell peppers, preferably yellow or orange

Stuffing Option 1
1½ teaspoons olive oil
1½ tablespoons balsamic vinegar
1 clove garlic, minced
¾ pound tomatoes of choice, seeded and coarsely chopped
1 cup fresh mozzarella cheese cubes
½ cup fresh basil leaves cut into strips
Salt and ground black pepper to taste

Stuffing Option 2
1 tablespoon olive oil
¾ pound tomatoes of choice, seeded and coarsely chopped
1 cup feta cheese cubes
½ cup quartered, pitted kalamata olives
Fresh or dried oregano to taste
Salt and ground black pepper to taste

1. Preheat the oven to 375°F.
2. Cut the peppers in half lengthwise and remove the seeds and ribs. Set aside.
3. Combine all the ingredients for either filling in a bowl and stuff each pepper with the filling.
4. Place in a greased baking dish and bake until the peppers are tender, about 40 minutes.

Option 1: 4 servings. Per serving: 128 calories, 7 g protein, 9 g carbohydrate, 8 g fat, 2 g fiber

Option 2: 4 servings. Per serving: 160 calories, 6 g protein, 6 g carbohydrate, 13 g fat, 2 g fiber

Cumin Grilled Zucchini
with Tomato-Corn Salsa

From *Dishing with Kathy Casey:* "These vegetables can be served hot or at room temperature. It's a great dish to take to a summer barbecue or picnic potluck."

Tomato-Corn Salsa
¾ cup finely chopped ripe tomatoes
1 cup (about 1 ear) fresh sweet corn kernels
¼ cup finely chopped red onion
1 fresh jalapeño chile pepper, seeded and finely chopped
       (wear plastic gloves when handling)
1 tablespoon red wine vinegar
2 tablespoons olive oil
2 tablespoons chopped fresh cilantro
¾ teaspoon salt
¼ teaspoon ground cumin

Zucchini
1 tablespoon olive oil
1 teaspoon ground cumin
½ teaspoon salt
¼ teaspoon ground black pepper
3 medium zucchini (about 1¼ pounds)
Sour cream

1. To make the salsa, in a large bowl, mix the tomatoes, corn, onion, jalapeño pepper, vinegar, oil, cilantro, salt, and cumin together well. Some jalapeño peppers are hotter than others, so try a little piece before mixing it all in, and then adjust the amount as needed for the desired spiciness.

2. Get the coals going for a very hot grill.

3. To make the zucchini, in a large bowl, mix together the oil, cumin, salt, and pepper. Cut the zucchini in half lengthwise and add them to the bowl. Rub the oil mixture over the zucchini, making sure they are coated well.

4. Place the zucchini over very hot coals and grill for 2 to 3 minutes on each side to mark the zucchini nicely. Cook until just done. Depending on how hot the grill is and how done you like your vegetables, the total cooking time can vary from 4 to 10 minutes.

5. Serve the zucchini topped with the salsa and a dollop or squiggle of sour cream.

4 servings. Per serving: 185 calories, 4 g protein, 15 g carbohydrate, 14 g fat, 3 g fiber

19

Soups

Soup is wonderful stuff, true comfort food. But if you read the labels on the soup cans in your grocery store, you'll discover that most canned soups are loaded with starch. Rice, noodles, potatoes, legumes, or cornstarch thickeners—it's hard to find a soup that doesn't have at least one starchy ingredient.

Luckily, soup is easy to make. You'll be dazzled by how much better it is than canned, frozen, or especially (ugh) dried soup. You know how much better Mom's homemade chocolate chip cookies are than the bagged ones? That's how much better homemade soup is than canned.

About Broth

Most soups begin with broth, and the better your broth, the better your soup will be. It is worthwhile to try several brands of packaged broth to find the one you like the best—we think Kitchen Basics brand is good, and it's made from reassuringly real ingredients.

Better yet, make your own broth. It's so easy it's ridiculous. Here's how to always have homemade broth on hand.

- Save all your chicken bones in a plastic grocery sack in the freezer. You can save steak bones in another sack, to make beef broth. It doesn't matter if all the meat is gone; stark naked bones will make great broth.

- When you have a sackful of bones, dump them into your biggest nonreactive kettle (such as stainless steel). Cover them with water and add a teaspoon or two of salt and about ¼ cup of vinegar—any kind. Stick it on a back burner, set it on low, and let it simmer until the water's cooked down by about a third.

- Strain it, dump the bones in the trash, and you've got far better broth than any you can buy. If you have more than you can use right away, freeze your broth in airtight containers. Having a couple of quarts of broth in the freezer is like money in the bank!

Soup's On!

If your weeknights are busy, make a double or triple batch of soup over the weekend. Then you can just ladle some into a bowl, zap it in the microwave oven, and supper's ready!

Here are some popular low-glycemic-load soups you'll see in cookbooks and restaurant menus, as well as some recipes for my favorites.

- **Gazpacho:** This chilled summertime favorite is made with tomatoes, bell peppers, onions, and cucumbers.
- **Borscht:** The Russian classic has many variations, made with beets, beef, tomatoes, onions, cabbage, and seasonings. It's delicious hot or chilled, topped with a dollop of sour cream.
- **Hot and sour soup:** Chances are, you'll find this bracing soup with pork, mushrooms, and tofu on the menu in your favorite Chinese restaurant or in many cookbooks.
- **Garden vegetable:** You can make this nutritious favorite with chicken, beef, or vegetable broth and all kinds of vegetables; just pluck out the potatoes.
- **Bouillabaisse:** This French favorite is a hearty fish soup that combines shellfish, fish fillets, bacon, and vegetables.

Pho

Say "fuh." This beef noodle soup is Vietnamese comfort food, and it's wonderful. Sheer bliss.

>   6 cups beef broth
>   1 cinnamon stick, 3" long
>   2 whole star anise (see note)
>   ½" fresh ginger, thinly sliced
>   10 ounces beef sirloin, well trimmed
>   14 ounces traditional shirataki noodles
>   1 teaspoon chili garlic paste, or to taste
>   ¼ cup fish sauce (nuoc mam or nam pla)
>   1 cup mung bean sprouts
>   4 scallions, including the crisp greens, thinly sliced
>   ¼ cup chopped fresh cilantro
>   ¼ cup chopped fresh basil
>   1 lime, cut into wedges

1. Pour the broth into a kettle or large saucepan and put it over high heat. Add the cinnamon, star anise, and ginger. Bring the broth to a simmer and turn the heat down so the liquid keeps simmering while you do the rest.

2. Trim any fat off the beef and slice it as thinly as possible, across the grain. (It's easier to slice meat thinly if it's partly frozen.)

3. Put the noodles into a strainer and rinse well. Use kitchen shears to snip across them several times in different directions.

4. When your broth has been simmering for 15 minutes, you can, if you like, skim out the spices with a slotted spoon, but it's not strictly necessary. Now add the beef and stir to keep the slices from sticking together. Add the noodles and stir in the chili garlic paste and fish sauce. Let the whole thing continue simmering for 5 minutes or so, until the beef's cooked through.

5. Add the bean sprouts and cook for another minute or so. Then ladle into bowls, top each bowl with scallions, cilantro, and basil, and serve with a wedge of lime to squeeze into it.

3 servings. Per serving: 423 calories, 42 g protein, 24 g carbohy-drate, 18 g fat, 6 g fiber

Note: Star anise is available at Asian markets and often in the international food aisle of big grocery stores. It comes whole, not ground, and it really is shaped like a star. Store star anise in a jar with a tight lid.

Curried Coconut Cream of Chicken Soup

So simple and so good! If you don't have coconut milk in the house, cream will do. But why not keep coconut milk in the house?

>   6 cups chicken broth
>   12 ounces boneless, skinless chicken breast (about
>   3 breasts)
>   3 tablespoons curry powder
>   2 teaspoons chicken bouillon concentrate
>   ½ tablespoon butter
>   ⅓ cup sliced almonds
>   1 can (13½ ounces) coconut milk
>   Guar or xanthan (optional)

1. Put the broth in a big saucepan over medium-high heat and let it start warming as you finely chop the chicken breast. Stir the chicken into the broth. (If you just dump it in, it will sit in the bottom of the pan and congeal back into a big lump.) Stir in the curry powder and bouillon concentrate and keep it cooking.

2. In a small skillet, melt the butter over medium heat. Add the almonds and stir them in the butter until they're a nice golden color. Remove from the heat.

3. Stir the coconut milk into the soup. Let the whole thing cook for another minute or two. Thicken it a bit with your guar or xanthan shaker if you like. Serve with the toasted almonds on top.

5 servings. Per serving: 394 calories, 25 g protein, 10 g carbohydrate, 30 g fat, 4 g fiber

Easy Chicken Gumbo

When I found frozen gumbo mix in my grocery store, this became inevitable. Feel free to use shrimp instead, or half shrimp, half chicken, or even andouille sausage.

> 2 slices bacon, finely chopped
> 1 pound frozen gumbo mix vegetables
> 2 quarts chicken broth
> 1 pound boneless, skinless chicken breasts, thighs, or both
> 1 can (14½ ounces) diced tomatoes
> 2 teaspoons hot-pepper sauce, or to taste
> 1 clove garlic, crushed
> ½ teaspoon dried thyme
> ½ teaspoon ground black pepper
> ¼ teaspoon ground red pepper, or to taste

1. Put your soup kettle or a good, big saucepan over medium heat. Put the bacon in the kettle and start it browning.

2. When the bacon is just starting to get crisp, add the frozen gumbo mix—no need to thaw it first—and the chicken broth.

3. Cut the chicken into ½" cubes and stir it into the soup (don't just dump it in, or it will sink to the bottom of the pot and cook together into a big lump). Stir in the tomatoes, hot-pepper sauce, garlic, thyme, black pepper, and red pepper, bring the whole thing to a simmer, and let it cook until the veggies are tender.

5 servings. Per serving: 252 calories, 31 g protein, 16 g carbohydrate, 6 g fat, 2 g fiber

Grandma's Chicken Soup

Of all the grains, barley has the lowest glycemic load. It's still starchy as heck, of course, so you can't eat bowls and bowls of it. But in a soup like this it's fine—and tastes great.

> 2 quarts chicken broth
> ¼ cup barley
> 1 large carrot, sliced
> 1 medium onion, finely chopped
> 1 large rib celery, finely chopped
> 1 teaspoon poultry seasoning
> 2 bay leaves
> 12 ounces boneless, skinless chicken thighs, finely chopped

1. Put your soup kettle or biggest saucepan over medium heat and dump in the chicken broth. Add the barley and get the whole thing heating.

2. After the broth has warmed up, toss in the carrot, onion, and celery, along with the poultry seasoning and bay leaves.

3. Cut your chicken into ½" cubes and stir it into the soup. (Don't just dump it in. It'll cook together into a big lump in the bottom of the pot. Stir it in.)

4. Let the whole thing simmer until the barley's cooked—maybe 40 minutes.

6 servings. Per serving: 227 calories, 17 g protein, 10 g carbohydrate, 12 g fat, 2 g fiber

Note: You could substitute a package of fettuccine-width tofu shirataki noodles for the barley, for chicken noodle soup.

Oyster Bisque

Elegant and rich.

> 2 tablespoons butter
> 1 cup finely chopped celery
> 1 cup finely chopped onion
> 1 pound shucked raw oysters
> Bottled clam juice, if needed
> 1 pinch saffron threads
> ¼ teaspoon guar or xanthan
> ¾ teaspoon ground coriander
> ½ teaspoon salt, or to taste
> ⅛ teaspoon ground red pepper
> 3 cups milk or half-and-half
> ¼ cup chopped parsley

1. In a large saucepan over medium-low heat, melt the butter and start cooking the celery and onion, stirring frequently; you want them to soften, not brown.

2. Meanwhile, put a strainer over a bowl and drain the oysters. Pour the liquid that drains off the oysters into a measuring cup. You want 1 cup. If you're a little short, make up the difference with bottled clam juice. For the moment, pop the oysters back into the fridge.

3. When the onion is translucent and the celery softening, add the oyster liquid and the saffron. Bring to a simmer, cover, and cook for 20 to 30 minutes.

4. If you have a stick blender, you can puree your vegetables right in the pan. If you don't, you'll have to transfer the mixture to your blender or food processor (with the S blade in place). Whichever device you use, add the guar or xanthan, coriander, salt, and ground red pepper and puree them into the celery-onion mixture. Add the milk or half-and-half and puree again.

(continued)

5. Return the mixture to the pan (if you took it out in the first place). Turn the heat to low. Heat slowly—milk or half-and-half scorches easily. While it's heating, pull the oysters out of the fridge and coarsely chop them.

6. When your soup is simmering, stir in the oysters and parsley. Let it simmer for another 3 to 5 minutes, until the oysters are cooked through, and serve.

4 servings. Per serving: 264 calories, 15 g protein, 18 g carbohydrate, 15 g fat, 1 g fiber

Seriously Simple Southwestern Sausage Soup

The name says it all! Feel free to use turkey sausage if you prefer.

    1 pound bulk pork sausage
    1 tablespoon ground cumin
    1 teaspoon dried oregano
    6 cups chicken broth
    1 jar (16 ounces) salsa
    1 can (15 ounces) black soybeans

1. In a kettle or big saucepan, brown and crumble the sausage. When it's cooked through, drain off any grease.

2. Add the cumin, oregano, broth, salsa, and soybeans, bring to a simmer, and serve.

5 servings. Per serving: 456 calories, 18 g protein, 8 g carbohydrate, 39 g fat, 2 g fiber

Super-Chunky Slow-Cooker Vegetable-Beef Soup

This really is super-chunky—more meat and vegetables than broth. If you have a really big slow cooker, you could double the broth in this recipe and still have a good, chunky soup.

  1 quart beef broth
  1 medium turnip, finely chopped
  1 medium carrot, sliced
  1 medium onion, finely chopped
  1 cup frozen crosscut green beans
  1 cup frozen peas
  1 can (15 ounces) diced tomatoes
  1 pound boneless beef chuck, well trimmed and cut into
      ½" cubes
  1 medium rib celery, including leaves, finely chopped
  2 bay leaves
  Salt and ground black pepper to taste

1. Pour the broth into your slow cooker and place the root vegetables—the turnip, carrot, and onion—at the bottom. Add the green beans, peas, tomatoes, beef, celery, and bay leaves.

2. Cover and cook on low for 8 to 10 hours. Add salt and pepper and serve.

5 servings. Per serving: 311 calories, 26 g protein, 19 g carbohydrate, 15 g fat, 3 g fiber

Red Bell Pepper Soup Topped with Sour Cream

Red bell pepper soup is mainstream gourmet when flavored with summer savory but suddenly becomes Mexican gourmet when you add oregano. Either way, be sure to garnish the warm soup with chilled sour cream to add richness and balance the textures and flavors.

> 1 cup finely chopped onion
> 1 tablespoon unrefined safflower oil
> 1 jar (15 ounces) roasted yellow and red peppers, or
>   1 yellow and 1 red fresh bell pepper, roasted,
>   trimmed, and chopped
> 1 medium tomato
> 2 cups chicken broth, divided
> ¼ teaspoon dried summer savory
> Salt and ground black pepper to taste
> Sour cream for garnish

1. In a small skillet, cook the onion in the oil over medium heat, stirring frequently, until softened and translucent, about 5 minutes.

2. Put the roasted peppers, tomato, and onion in a food processor fitted with a metal blade. Puree with a splash of the chicken broth.

3. Transfer the puree to a saucepan. Add the rest of the broth and the summer savory. Season with salt and black pepper to taste.

4. Bring the soup almost to a boil and reduce the heat to low. Cover the pot and simmer for 15 minutes. Ladle the soup into individual bowls and garnish each serving with a dollop of sour cream.

4 servings. Per serving: 129 calories, 5 g protein, 12 g carbohydrate, 8 g fat, 2 g fiber

20

Poultry

Do you love chicken? We never tire of the stuff. Chicken is great simply roasted, and it also lends itself to endless variations. It's reliably cheap. The boneless, skinless stuff is even quick to cook.

Too, chicken is a crowd pleaser. Kids like it, most diets allow it, and it doesn't run afoul (a fowl? sorry) of most religious dietary laws. Truly, it's hard to go wrong with chicken—especially when you have a bunch of great ways to cook it!

Chicken Dishes

Chicken has become a mainstay of the American diet because it is less expensive than other main-course options and endlessly versatile. It can be served hot or cold and prepared in dozens of different ways.

- **Coq au vin:** This French classic is a chicken stew slowly simmered with mushrooms, onions, garlic, herbs, and red wine until the meat falls away from the bone.
- **Chicken fricassee:** This delicate, creamy dish combines chicken and vegetables—a longtime favorite on American dinner tables.

Simple Roasted Chicken

You can roast any cut-up chicken (skin on, bone in) this way. Always roast extra. Then you'll have cold chicken in the fridge for chicken salad or just to eat on its own.

Turn your oven to 375°F or 400°F. Sprinkle the chicken with a little something to season it—you can use:

Good ol' salt and ground black pepper
Barbecue rub
Cajun seasoning
Creole seasoning
Jerk seasoning

If you think about it ahead of time, put your chicken in a resealable plastic bag and pour in enough bottled vinaigrette dressing to coat it. Seal the bag, pressing out the air as you go, turn it to coat the chicken, then throw the bag into the fridge. When it's time to cook, just pour off the dressing and roast.

Or you can pull back the skin and put a few fresh herbs underneath it—sage, oregano, thyme, and marjoram are all good.

However you season your chicken, arrange it in a roasting pan. Slide it into the oven and let it roast for 45 minutes at 400°F or about an hour at 375°F. Baste it once or twice during that time with the drippings in the bottom of the pan. It's done when it's brown and crisp all over.

- **Chicken parmigiana:** This Italian-American dish combines lightly breaded chicken cutlets with tomato sauce and Parmesan and mozzarella cheeses. (Substitute eggplant for chicken for a vegetarian version of this dish.)

We've also included a recipe for using up leftover turkey and one for adding family-pleasing flavor to the ground turkey.

Ginger-Sesame Glazed Chicken

This roasted chicken has a great Asian glaze.

> 1 tablespoon grated fresh ginger
> ½ cup soy sauce
> ¼ cup lime juice
> 1 tablespoon minced garlic
> 1 tablespoon dark sesame oil
> 1 tablespoon honey
> 2 tablespoons Splenda
> 3 pounds chicken pieces

1. In a small bowl, mix together the ginger, soy sauce, lime juice, garlic, oil, honey, and Splenda. Place the chicken in a big resealable plastic bag or a glass dish and pour the ginger-soy mixture over it. If using a bag, press the air out and seal, then turn over to coat the chicken. If using a dish, turn the chicken over a couple of times to coat. Either way, refrigerate your chicken and let it marinate for at least an hour or two. If marinating in a dish, turn it over at least once during the marinating time.

2. Preheat your oven to 375°F. Pour the marinade off the chicken into a bowl and reserve. Lay your chicken skin side up in a roasting pan.

3. Roast for 75 minutes, basting with the reserved marinade every 15 to 20 minutes; do not baste for at least the final 10 minutes of cooking time.

5 servings. Per serving: 462 calories, 36 g protein, 9 g carbohydrate, 31 g fat, trace fiber

Lemon-Lime Chicken

The tangy marinade enhances the flavor of the chicken itself.

> **3 pounds cut-up chicken, light meat or dark or any combination**
> **¼ cup lemon juice**
> **¼ cup lime juice**
> **¼ cup dry white wine**
> **¼ cup olive oil**
> **2 cloves garlic, crushed**
> **1 teaspoon salt or Vege-Sal**
> **⅛ teaspoon ground black pepper**
> **1 teaspoon hot-pepper sauce**
> **¼ teaspoon dried thyme**

1. Put the chicken in a big resealable plastic bag or a bowl. Mix together the lemon juice, lime juice, wine, oil, garlic, salt or Vege-Sal, black pepper, hot-pepper sauce, and thyme and pour it into the bag. Seal the bag, pressing out the air as you go. Toss the bag into the fridge and let the whole thing marinate for at least a few hours; all day is great. (If you think of it, flip the bag over whenever you stick your head in the fridge, but it's not essential.)

2. When it's time to cook, preheat your oven to 400°F. Retrieve your bag from the fridge and pour off the marinade into a bowl. Arrange the chicken in a roasting pan.

3. Roast for about 45 minutes, basting a few times with the reserved marinade. When your chicken is well browned and the juices run clear when you pierce the chicken to the bone, it's done.

6 servings. Per serving: 427 calories, 29 g protein, 3 g carbohydrate, 32 g fat, trace fiber

Cashew-Crusted Chicken

Good as is; even better with the Apricot-Mustard Dressing on page 213 as a dipping sauce.

> 2½ pounds boneless, skinless chicken breasts
> 1 cup raw cashew pieces (see note)
> ½ teaspoon salt or Vege-Sal
> ¼ teaspoon garlic powder
> ¼ teaspoon onion powder
> ½ teaspoon curry powder
> Pinch of ground red pepper
> 2 tablespoons butter

1. Pound each chicken breast out to ½" thick by putting them in a resealable plastic bag one at a time and whacking with a heavy, blunt object. Cut into 6 equal portions.

2. Put the cashews in your food processor with the S blade in place and add the salt or Vege-Sal, garlic powder, onion powder, curry powder, and ground red pepper. Pulse until the cashews are chopped medium-fine—you want some texture left. Spread this mixture on a big plate.

3. One piece at a time, press both sides of each of the pieces of chicken breast in the seasoned cashews.

4. Spray your biggest skillet with cooking spray and put it over medium heat. Melt the butter and cook the chicken for about 5 minutes per side, stirring frequently, until golden and crisp on the outside and done through. Serve immediately.

6 servings. Per serving: 383 calories, 46 g protein, 6 g carbohydrate, 19 g fat, 1 g fiber

Note: You can use whole raw cashews for this recipe, but at my health food store raw cashew pieces are less than half the price of whole cashews. So I buy the pieces.

Orange Soy Chicken Asparagus Stir-Fry

Most stir-fry recipes have a low glycemic load as long as you don't serve them over rice. The orange makes this one citrusy fresh, yet it isn't enough to spike your blood sugar.

> 1 orange
> 2 tablespoons soy sauce
> ½ clove garlic
> 2 teaspoons Splenda or sugar
> 12 ounces boneless, skinless chicken breast
> ½ pound asparagus
> 1 medium onion, sliced
> 1 tablespoon coconut oil or peanut oil

1. Grate the peel of the orange and squeeze its juice. In a mixing bowl, combine both with the soy sauce, garlic, and Splenda or sugar.

2. Cube the chicken breast and put it in the bowl with the orange juice mixture. Toss to make sure all the cubes are coated. Let this sit for at least 30 minutes.

3. Meanwhile, snap the ends off the asparagus pieces where they break naturally. Cut the pieces on the diagonal into ½" lengths. Peel the onion and cut it into half rounds about ¼" thick.

4. Put a big skillet or wok over the highest heat. Fish the chicken out of its marinade with a fork and put it on a plate by the stove, along with the veggies. Reserve the marinade.

5. When the pan is good and hot, add the oil. When the oil's hot, throw in the chicken. Stir-fry until all the pink is gone.

6. Scoop the chicken out and put it back in the bowl with the marinade. If the pan needs more oil, add just a touch more. Throw in the asparagus and onion and stir-fry until tender-crisp—the asparagus should be brilliant emerald green.

7. Add the cooked chicken and the marinade and stir it all together. Stir-fry for another few minutes and serve.

2 servings. Per serving: 338 calories, 41 g protein, 17 g carbohydrate, 12 g fat, 4 g fiber

Blue Cheese Walnut Pesto Chicken with Noodles

Awfully fancy, considering that you can put it together in 20 minutes flat!

16 ounces tofu shirataki noodles, fettuccine style
¼ cup chicken broth
1 tablespoon butter, divided
¼ cup chopped walnuts
8 ounces boneless, skinless chicken thighs or breasts
¼ cup finely chopped onion
1 clove garlic, crushed
⅓ cup half-and-half
2 tablespoons jarred pesto sauce
5½ ounces crumbled blue cheese, divided

1. Open the shirataki noodles and toss them into a strainer. Rinse well. Now put them in a bowl and stir in the chicken broth. Let this sit for about 30 minutes or even all day.

2. Melt a teaspoon of the butter in a small skillet over medium-low heat and stir the walnuts in it until they smell toasty. Remove from the heat and set aside.

3. Cut the chicken into ½" chunks. Melt the rest of the butter in your big, heavy skillet over medium heat and start the chicken and onion cooking in it, stirring frequently. While that's happening, put the shirataki and broth in a small saucepan and set over a burner to warm.

4. When all the pink is gone from the chicken and the onion is translucent, stir in the garlic, half-and-half, and pesto. Now add all but a couple of tablespoons of the blue cheese. Stir until the cheese is melted and the sauce is thick.

5. Using tongs or a slotted spoon, lift the noodles out of their broth and pile them on 3 plates or bowls. Divide the chicken mixture and sauce among them. Top each with a third of the reserved blue cheese and walnuts and serve.

3 servings. Per serving: 456 calories, 27 g protein, 6 g carbohydrate, 36 g fat, 1 g fiber

Turkey Meat Loaf

Ground turkey is inexpensive, but it's often bland. This turkey meat loaf is bursting with flavor!

> **1 medium carrot**
> **1 medium rib celery**
> **1 medium onion**
> **1 small apple**
> **2 pounds ground turkey**
> **1 tablespoon poultry seasoning**
> **2 tablespoons Worcestershire sauce**
> **2 teaspoons salt or Vege-Sal**
> **½ cup oat bran**
> **1 egg**

1. Preheat the oven to 350°F.

2. Using the shredding disk, run the carrot, celery, onion, and apple through your food processor. You'll end up with some unshredded produce atop the disk. Chop that stuff up with a knife or grate it on your box grater and throw it in too.

3. Add all the shredded stuff into a big mixing bowl and add the turkey, poultry seasoning, Worcestershire sauce, salt or Vege-Sal, oat bran, and egg. Using clean hands, mush everything together until it's very well blended.

4. Pack the mixture into a loaf pan and bake for 45 minutes. Let sit for 10 minutes before serving.

8 servings. Per serving: 216 calories, 22 g protein, 10 g carbohydrate, 10 g fat, 2 g fiber

Smoked Turkey, Sun-Dried Tomato, and Yellow Bell Pepper Pizza

If you don't have a yellow bell pepper, a green or red one will do; your pizza will still be ultraspecial.

1 yellow bell pepper, thinly sliced
½ medium onion, thinly sliced
1 clove garlic, crushed
1 tablespoon olive oil, plus a little for brushing the tortillas
¾ pound sliced smoked turkey breast
¾ cup drained oil-packed sun-dried tomatoes
2 tablespoons jarred pesto sauce
2 large low-carb tortillas
1½ cups shredded mozzarella cheese

1. Preheat the oven to 425°F.
2. In your big, heavy skillet over medium heat, start cooking the bell pepper, onion, and garlic in the oil, stirring frequently.
3. Cut the turkey breast slices into 1" squares—just cut through all the slices at once. With the S blade in place, plunk them into your food processor. Add the sun-dried tomatoes and the pesto. Pulse until everything is chopped to a medium consistency.
4. Lay a tortilla on a baking sheet. Brush it lightly with a little of the oil. Now spread half the turkey mixture on top. Cover that with half the pepper-onion mixture and top that with ¾ cup shredded mozzarella. Repeat with the second tortilla and the rest of the ingredients.
5. Bake for about 10 minutes, or until the cheese is melted and getting a few golden spots. Cut into quarters to serve.

4 servings. Per serving: 450 calories, 34 g protein, 19 g carbohydrate, 28 g fat, 9 g fiber

Cranberry Salsa

Not a chicken recipe, but a great way to liven up simple grilled or roasted chicken.

>1 jalapeño chile pepper—2 if you like your salsa really
>hot! (wear plastic gloves when handling)
>½ large orange
>½ medium red onion, cut into chunks
>12 ounces fresh cranberries
>¾ cup Splenda or sugar, or to taste
>3 tablespoons lime juice
>¼ teaspoon salt
>¼ teaspoon ground cinnamon
>½ cup chopped fresh cilantro

1. Split the jalapeño pepper down the middle and remove the seeds, ribs, and stem. Put it in your food processor with the S blade in place.

2. Grate the peel of your orange and reserve. Then seed the orange and put the flesh in the processor with the jalapeño pepper. Add the onion. Pulse the food processor until everything is chopped to a medium consistency.

3. Add the cranberries and pulse until they're chopped to a medium consistency. Transfer the mixture to a glass, plastic, stainless steel, or enamel bowl.

4. Stir in the Splenda or sugar, lime juice, salt, cinnamon, and cilantro. Chill for an hour or two to let the flavors marry, then serve with any poultry—or with pork, for that matter.

8 servings. Per serving: 40 calories, trace protein, 10 g carbohydrate, trace fat, 2 g fiber

Note: Fresh cranberries are one of the few fruits that are still strictly seasonal; they're available only in the autumn and winter. But they freeze beautifully. Just buy a few extra bags and throw them in your freezer, and you can make cranberry salsa year-round.

21

Beef

Beef draws a lot of fire. Health-conscious people shun it or eat it with a sneaking sense of guilt. But it's time to get over your beef phobia. Beef is darned nutritious stuff. Comparing 6 ounces of beef flank steak with an equal portion of boneless, skinless chicken breast, the beef has more potassium, iron, thiamin, riboflavin, and folic acid and vastly more zinc and vitamin B_{12}—all for a big 66 extra calories. Both are equally devoid of carbohydrate. Very simply, beef is good for you.

What about beef fat? Isn't it terribly saturated? Half of the fat in beef is unsaturated. Further, half of the saturated fat is in the form of stearic acid, a saturated fat that has the same effect on blood fats as olive oil does—which is to say, it lowers your bad cholesterol and raises your good cholesterol. Stop worrying.

Better, buy grass-fed beef. Yes, it's pricey, and you'll probably have to go out of your way to find it, but grass-fed beef is on a par with salmon for healthy omega-3 fats. It's also better for the environment.

There's nothing like tucking into a big steak, with a crisp salad on the side and a big glass of red wine, to make you think, "What diet?!" As long as you skip the baked potato and Texas toast, you are now free to think of steak as a healthy dinner.

The same goes for a big pot of chili, a grilled burger, or a slab of prime rib!

Red Meat Mainstays

Although we know now that meat is not the problem, along the way you might have lost interest in learning about new ways to prepare it. Chances are, your meat dishes have remained somewhat unimaginative over the years. Of course, a grilled steak with nothing but salt and pepper for seasoning will always be a favorite, but there are many exciting ways to enhance the flavor and texture of meat. You can also experiment with dry rubs, marinades, flavored butters, glazes, salsas, and classic sauces like Madeira and béarnaise. Here are some popular ways of enhancing meat dishes, followed by several of my favorite meat recipes.

- **Boeuf bourguignon:** The classic French version of braised beef stew is prepared with bacon, mushrooms, carrots, pearl onions, and red wine. It's a winter favorite.
- **London broil:** This is flank steak quickly grilled or broiled over high heat and thinly sliced across the grain. Experiment with different marinades, and throw leftovers into a salad with lettuce, mushrooms, red onion, and crumbled blue cheese.
- **Meat loaf:** A family favorite in American homes for decades, this is comfort food without the carbs (except for an inconsequential amount of bread crumbs).
- **Chili:** This spicy mix of beef and seasonings made from chile peppers originated in Texas, but options for preparing it extend far beyond the original "con carne" version. You can make it with any kind of meat or poultry.
- **Kebabs:** Thread meat, poultry, or fish onto skewers, alternating with pieces of vegetables. Brush with olive oil or marinade and grill.
- **Barbecue:** Now beloved by Americans in all parts of the country, barbecue dishes can be made in the oven or on the grill in endless ways, including beef brisket, country-style pork ribs, and chicken slathered in your favorite sauce.

Burger Basics

Other countries include ground meat in their cuisines, but America has elevated it to the status of a national dish. I am here to defend the venerable hamburger patty. It's the hamburger's pals that cause the trouble—the bun, the fries, and the soda or shake.

If you eat a quarter-pound burger with cheese, a supersize order of fries, and a giganto sugared soda, you'll get more than 1,600 calories, which—let's face it—is part of the problem right there. But just 450 of those calories come from fat, just 28 percent. Our hypothetical fast-food meal is a perfect illustration of the Glycemic Load Diet's simple rule—knock out the starch and the sugared beverages and you'll be fine.

So, eat hamburgers! Just eat 'em with a fork, topping a salad, or wrapped in lettuce, rather than on a bun. And skip the fries and the liquid candy. (If you can't resist the fries, stay out of the fast-food joints!)

We like ground chuck best for burgers. It has a great lean-to-fat ratio and a great flavor. When ground chuck goes on sale, we buy 20 pounds or more, make it into 6-ounce patties (a little bigger than a third of a pound), and freeze them. Sound like too much work? Look in your grocery store's freezer case. Very likely they have premade

- **Curries:** Experiment with this exotic import for a different, delicious taste sensation. There are endless varieties; you can make curry with lamb, chicken, shrimp, or vegetables. The flavors will be so intriguing, you won't miss eating the rice that often accompanies it.

hamburger patties, which are a terrific convenience food. Just read the label to make sure they have no starchy fillers. (If the burgers are 100 percent beef, the label is likely to boast of it in bold print.)

Whether you make your own or buy premade patties, it's up to you whether you want to pan-broil your burgers, run them under the broiler, or throw them on your electric tabletop grill. However you cook them, they're quick and easy protein.

But a bunless burger sounds sort of . . . well, plain. You can top it with the usual ketchup, mustard, and pickles if you like. But there are plenty of other things to do to a burger. Try:

- A sprinkle of barbecue rub—plus barbecue sauce if you like
- Melted mozzarella and pizza sauce
- Pepper Jack cheese and salsa
- Blue cheese and finely chopped red onion
- Cooked onions, mushrooms, or both
- Crumbled feta and chopped olives
- Mayonnaise seasoned with crushed garlic and snipped herbs

Joe

This is how we currently make "Joe's Special," a venerable recipe that apparently started in San Francisco. Feel free to play with this; it's hard to make a bad batch of Joe. The immutable basics are ground beef, onion, garlic, spinach, and eggs. But you can use more or less meat, more or fewer eggs. You can leave out the cheese or add more. If you have some mushrooms hanging around the house, they'd be good in here. Some people add a shot of Worcestershire, others a dash or two of hot-pepper sauce, still others a little oregano or nutmeg or even coriander.

> 1½ pounds ground chuck or round
> 1 large onion, chopped
> 3 cloves garlic, crushed
> 10 ounces frozen chopped spinach, thawed and drained
>   well (see note)
> 6 eggs, beaten
> Salt and ground black pepper to taste
> ⅓ cup grated fresh Parmesan cheese

1. Put your big, heavy skillet over medium heat and throw in your ground chuck or round. Start it browning and crumbling.

2. When some fat has cooked out of your meat, throw in the onion and garlic. Keep cooking (and crumbling the meat) until all the pink is gone from the meat and the onion is soft and translucent. Tilt the pan, scoop the meat-and-onion mixture to the top of the slope, and use a big spoon to spoon out as much grease as you can.

3. Now stir in the thawed spinach and the eggs and keep stirring until the eggs are set. Season with salt and pepper, sprinkle the Parmesan over everything, and serve.

6 servings. Per serving: 406 calories, 29 g protein, 5 g carbohydrate, 29 g fat, 2 g fiber

Note: Spinach can hold a lot of water! Dump it into a strainer and press it with the back of a spoon. Or—this is easier—use clean hands and squeeze it hard.

Jersey Girl Chili

So good! It's the faint Italian accent that gives this chili its New Jersey attitude.

    12 ounces mild Italian sausage
    1½ pounds ground chuck
    2 medium onions, chopped
    2 cloves garlic, crushed
    1 can (14½ ounces) diced tomatoes
    1 can (8 ounces) tomato sauce
    ¼ cup dry red wine
    2 tablespoons lemon juice
    ⅓ cup chili powder
    3 tablespoons ground cumin
    1 tablespoon dried basil
    1 tablespoon dried oregano
    1½ teaspoons salt or Vege-Sal
    1½ teaspoons ground black pepper
    1 teaspoon beef bouillon concentrate
    ¾ cup water
    1 can (15 ounces) black soybeans

1. Put your biggest skillet over medium heat and throw in the sausage and ground chuck. (If your sausage is in links, remove the casings so you can crumble it with the beef.) Brown and crumble the two together until cooked through. When the meat is done, drain off the fat.

2. Add the onions and garlic and continue cooking, stirring from time to time, until the onions have softened a little. Then simply add everything else, stirring carefully.

3. Turn the heat down and simmer for 40 to 45 minutes. Serve with a dollop of sour cream and a handful of shredded Cheddar cheese, if desired.

8 servings. Per serving: 441 calories, 24 g protein, 13 g carbohydrate, 33 g fat, 3 g fiber

Frenchified Meat Loaf

The recipe we adapted this from called for herbes de Provence, which I didn't have on hand. It also called for a lot more bread. So we made it this way, and it was wildly flavorful.

> **1 pound ground chuck**
> **½ pound bulk mild pork sausage**
> **2 slices low-carb whole grain bread, finely crumbed, or**
> **⅓ cup oat bran**
> **½ cup finely chopped onion**
> **1 clove garlic, minced**
> **¼ cup chopped parsley**
> **¼ cup dry red wine**
> **1 egg**
> **1 tablespoon Dijon or spicy brown mustard**
> **½ teaspoon dried savory**
> **½ teaspoon dried thyme**
> **¼ teaspoon ground rosemary**
> **½ teaspoon salt or 1 teaspoon Vege-Sal**
> **¼ teaspoon ground black pepper**

1. Preheat the oven to 350°F.

2. In a large bowl, mix the ground chuck, sausage, bread or oat bran, onion, garlic, parsley, wine, egg, mustard, savory, thyme, rosemary, salt or Vege-Sal, and black pepper. Use clean hands to squish them all together until they're really well mixed.

3. Now pack your meat loaf mixture into a loaf pan and bake for 50 to 60 minutes. Remove from the oven, drain the fat out of the pan, and let the loaf sit for 5 to 10 minutes before slicing and serving.

8 servings. Per serving: 304 calories, 16 g protein, 4 g carbohydrate, 24 g fat, 1 g fiber

Horseradish Sauce

Horseradish and beef are a classic combination. Spoon this over any steak you make.

> ¼ cup mayonnaise (we use light mayo because it's less
>   likely to "break" when it hits the hot steak)
> 2 tablespoons sour cream
> 1 scallion, including the crisp greens, minced
> 1 tablespoon prepared horseradish

Just mix together the mayonnaise, sour cream, scallion, and horseradish and spoon over steak.

6 servings. Per serving: 35 calories, trace protein, 1 g carbohydrate, 3 g fat, trace fiber

Fire Steak

But only a small fire. This won't burn your tastebuds off.

> ¼ cup hot-pepper sauce
> 3 tablespoons water
> 1 tablespoon Sucanat or 1 tablespoon Splenda and
>   ⅛ teaspoon blackstrap molasses (or the darkest
>   available)
> 1 pound beef rib eye or a good thick T-bone

1. Mix together the hot-pepper sauce, water, and Sucanat, or Splenda and molasses.

2. Pierce the steak all over with a fork. Put it in a resealable plastic bag and pour in the marinade. Seal the bag, pressing out the air as you go. Turn to coat the steak with the marinade. Throw the bag in the fridge and let it sit—all day if you can, but at least for an hour or two.

3. Now broil or grill the steak close to the heat until done to your taste and serve.

3 servings. Per serving: 278 calories, 31 g protein, 5 g carbohydrate, 14 g fat, trace fiber

Note: To turn an inexpensive chuck pot roast into a great, grillable steak, first make a double batch of this marinade. Then sprinkle your chuck steak with ½ teaspoon of meat tenderizer and pierce the steak all over. Flip and repeat on the other side, including another ½ teaspoon of meat tenderizer. Then marinate and grill as for Fire Steak. You can eat great on a budget!

Island Steak

These seasonings are classically Caribbean.

½ medium onion
1 jalapeño chile pepper (wear plastic gloves when
    handling)
¼ cup Splenda or Sucanat
¼ cup lime juice
¼ cup soy sauce
1 tablespoon grated fresh ginger
½ teaspoon ground allspice
½ teaspoon dried thyme
½ teaspoon paprika
3 cloves garlic
1½ teaspoons meat tenderizer
2 pounds boneless chuck roast, 1½"–2" thick

1. Throw the onion, jalapeño pepper, Splenda or Sucanat, lime juice, soy sauce, ginger, allspice, thyme, paprika, garlic, and meat tenderizer into your food processor with the S blade in place and pulse until the onion, jalapeño pepper, and garlic are quite finely chopped and you have a slurry.

2. Lay the chuck in a nonreactive dish (such as stainless steel or glass) and pierce it all over with a fork. Flip and pierce the other side too. Pour the marinade over the steak and flip it over again, making sure it's coated thoroughly on both sides. Now stash the whole thing in the fridge for several hours; overnight is even better.

3. Pull out your steak and pour off the marinade into a nonreactive pan. Broil the steak close to the flame until it's done to your liking; timing will depend on how thick it is. Meanwhile, bring the marinade to a boil and boil it hard for a few minutes to kill the raw meat germs. Serve with the steak.

6 servings. Per serving: 337 calories, 25 g protein, 5 g carbohydrate, 24 g fat, 1 g fiber

Beef and Bok Choy

Definitely worth going to the grocery store for the bok choy if you're not lucky enough to have green-thumbed neighbors.

½ pound boneless beef chuck
3 tablespoons soy sauce
½ teaspoon meat tenderizer
2 teaspoons dark sesame oil
1 clove garlic, minced
1 teaspoon honey or Splenda
¼ teaspoon chili garlic paste
2 tablespoons peanut oil
3 cups chopped bok choy (just quarter the heads
    lengthwise for baby bok choy)

1. Slice the beef across the grain as thinly as you can. (It helps to have the beef half frozen when you do this.)

2. In a nonreactive bowl (such as stainless steel or glass), mix together the soy sauce, meat tenderizer, sesame oil, garlic, honey or Splenda, and chili garlic paste. Add the beef slices and toss to coat with the soy mixture. Let sit for at least 30 minutes.

3. Put your wok or a big skillet over the highest heat. Add the peanut oil and let it get good and hot. Meanwhile, use a fork or tongs to lift the beef out of the marinade. Reserve the marinade.

4. Throw your drained beef slices into the skillet and stir-fry until the pink is gone. Add the bok choy and stir-fry for another minute or two. Pour the marinade over the stir-fry, stir-fry for another couple of minutes, and serve.

2 servings. Per serving: 437 calories, 21 g protein, 8 g carbohydrate, 36 g fat, 1 g fiber

Balsamic Slow-Cooker Short Ribs

Slow-cooker easy, but company good! Feel free to cut this recipe in half if you like. Personally, I love having leftovers in the fridge for a fast meal. Serve with Fauxtatoes (page 223) or Cauliflower-Potato Mash (page 224).

3 pounds meaty beef short ribs
1 onion, thinly sliced
8 ounces sliced mushrooms
1 clove garlic, crushed
¼ cup balsamic vinegar
¼ cup apple cider vinegar
2 tablespoons Sucanat, or 2 tablespoons Splenda and
    ½ teaspoon blackstrap molasses
1 tablespoon soy sauce
½ teaspoon mustard powder
1 tablespoon ketchup
½ teaspoon chili powder
1½ teaspoons beef bouillon concentrate
Guar or xanthan

1. Preheat your broiler.

2. Arrange the short ribs on the broiler rack and broil about 6" from the heat. You want to brown them for about 5 to 7 minutes per side.

3. Meanwhile, throw the onion, mushrooms, and garlic in the bottom of your slow cooker.

4. To make the sauce, mix together the vinegars, Sucanat or Splenda and molasses, soy sauce, mustard powder, ketchup, chili powder, and bouillon concentrate.

5. When the ribs are browned all over, place them on top of the onion and mushrooms. Now pour the sauce over the whole thing. Cover the slow cooker and set it on low. Let it all cook for 6 to 8 hours.

(continued)

6. When time's almost up, make your Fauxtatoes or Cauliflower-Potato Mash. Then uncover the slow cooker and use tongs to pull the ribs out onto 8 plates, next to the mash.

7. Use your guar or xanthan shaker to thicken up the sauce left in the pot, then spoon the sauce and veggies over the whole thing and serve.

8 servings. Per serving: 375 calories, 40 g protein, 5 g carbohydrate, 21 g fat, 1 g fiber

Mexican Pot Roast with Chili Powder Rub

Rubs are dry marinades—a great way to infuse an ordinary piece of meat with extraordinary flavor. In this recipe, chili powder is combined with garlic, oregano, and cinnamon to produce a dish with a decidedly south-of-the-border flavor. Serve with pinto beans, guacamole, and some chilled beer.

> 1 tablespoon chili powder
> 1 teaspoon dried oregano
> ½ teaspoon ground cinnamon
> 2 cloves garlic, minced
> Salt and ground black pepper to taste
> 2 pounds chuck or rump roast
> 2 tablespoons olive oil
> 2 medium onions
> 1 carrot
> 1 rib celery
> ½ cup red wine
> ½ cup homemade chicken, beef, or vegetable stock or
>   water

1. In a small bowl, combine the chili powder, oregano, cinnamon, garlic, salt, and pepper.

2. Sprinkle the spice mixture all over the roast and rub it into the meat. Refrigerate, covered, overnight.

3. Heat the oil over medium-high heat in a heavy pot with a tight-fitting lid. Put the meat in the pot and brown on all sides, about 10 minutes total.

4. Meanwhile, slice the onions and chop the carrot and celery into uniform small pieces.

5. Transfer the meat to a platter. Transfer the vegetables to the pot and cook over medium-high heat, stirring frequently, until softened and beginning to brown, about 10 minutes.

6. Add the wine and cook until most of the wine has evaporated. Scrape the bottom of the pot with a wooden spoon to prevent the vegetables from sticking.

(continued)

7. Add the stock and return the meat to the pot. Cover the pot and reduce the heat to very low. Cook the roast, turning occasionally, until very tender, 2 to 2½ hours, until a fork can easily pierce the meat and the juices run clear. Take care not to overcook the meat.

8. Transfer the roast to a serving platter and keep it warm. Skim the fat from the juices in the pot. Cook the juices, along with the mass of softened vegetables, on high, stirring and scraping the pot, until the juices reduce to a thick liquid. Slice the meat and serve the pot roast with the sauce and vegetables. This dish also makes an excellent leftover.

7 servings. Per serving: 351 calories, 45 g protein, 10 g carbohydrate, 13 g fat, 3 g fiber

Buffalo Burgers Stuffed with Cheddar Cheese

Just for a change, rustle up some buffalo meat. It's similar in flavor to beef but with slightly gamey overtones. In addition, free-range buffalo, like wild game, is a source of valuable omega-3 fatty acids. These burgers are sure to become a favorite around your household.

> **1 pound lean buffalo meat or 4 patties (4 ounces each) (see note)**
> **½ cup finely chopped onion**
> **¼ cup chopped parsley**
> **2 teaspoons Worcestershire sauce**
> **Salt and ground black pepper to taste**
> **1 cup loosely packed grated sharp Cheddar cheese**
> **Pickle relish or vinaigrette coleslaw for garnish (optional)**
> **4 low-carb tortillas (optional)**

1. Put the buffalo meat, onion, parsley, Worcestershire sauce, salt, and pepper in a large bowl and mix together.

2. Divide the meat into 4 equal portions. Shape each into a ball. Poke a deep hole into each ball, manually or with a spoon handle. Fill each with a quarter of the cheese. Press some meat over the opening to encase the cheese. With a spatula, flatten each ball into a patty ¾" thick.

3. Warm a grill pan over medium-high heat and cook the patties for about 5 minutes on each side for medium doneness.

4. Serve immediately, garnished with tart pickle relish or vinaigrette coleslaw. You can also fold each patty into a low-carb tortilla and add the usual hamburger toppings.

4 servings. Per serving: 264 calories, 38 g protein, 2 g carbohydrate, 10 g fat, 1 g fiber

Note: Buffalo meat patties are available frozen, and butchers can order select cuts from one of the growing number of producers.

22

Pork and Lamb

Pork is nothing if not controversial. It is the world's most popular meat, yet it is also the subject of religious taboos. Many people think of pork as an indulgence, even a guilty pleasure. This is a shame. Pork is indisputably delicious and also highly nutritious. Pork is a protein, of course, but it is also a surprisingly rich source of potassium and a good source of B vitamins. As for the much-maligned pork fat, it actually has more monounsaturates than saturates. Add to this the fact that pork is inexpensive! Enjoy pork guiltlessly as often as you like.

As for lamb, it is my favorite meat. I grew up loving lamb chops and roast leg of lamb, so it was a surprise to learn that many people have never even tried it. I hope you have, and if you haven't, I hope you will.

Before we get into the recipes, one idea was so simple we were reluctant to give it full recipe status: We adore pork shoulder steaks, simply pan broiled in a little olive oil and sprinkled with Creole seasoning or barbecue rub. With a big pile of coleslaw on the side, this is one of my favorite meals, and you can put it together in 15 minutes.

Lemon-Mustard Pork Chops

Warm, sunny flavors, and very quick and easy.

Salt and ground black pepper to taste
1½ pounds pork chops
2 tablespoons olive oil
½ cup chicken broth
1½ tablespoons dry vermouth
1 teaspoon dried thyme
1½ tablespoons Dijon or spicy brown mustard
1½ tablespoons lemon juice

1. Give your big, heavy skillet a shot of cooking spray. Put it over medium-high heat. While the skillet's heating, salt and pepper your chops lightly on both sides. When the skillet's hot, add the oil, slosh it around to cover the bottom of the skillet, then add the pork chops. Sear them until they're golden brown on both sides.

2. Add the broth, vermouth, and thyme to the skillet. Cover, turn the heat to medium-low, and let the chops simmer for 10 minutes, until cooked through but not dry.

3. Transfer the chops to plates. Turn the heat under the skillet to medium-high. Add the mustard and lemon juice and stir until the sauce is smooth and cooked down to the thickness of cream. Pour the sauce over the chops and serve.

4 servings. Per serving: 339 calories, 27 g protein, 1 g carbohydrate, 24 g fat, trace fiber

Pork Ribs Adobado

These ribs roast in the oven. They take time but are quite simple, and the results are so worth it.

> **2 teaspoons garlic powder**
> **1 tablespoon paprika**
> **1 teaspoon ground cumin**
> **1 teaspoon dried oregano**
> **1 teaspoon salt or Vege-Sal**
> **½ teaspoon ground black pepper**
> **3 pounds pork spareribs**
> **½ cup chicken broth or beer**
> **3 tablespoons olive oil**

1. Preheat the oven to 325°F.

2. In a small dish, stir together the garlic powder, paprika, cumin, oregano, salt or Vege-Sal, and black pepper. Transfer 1 tablespoon of the mixture to a cereal bowl and reserve.

3. Spray a roasting pan with cooking spray and throw in your slab of ribs. Sprinkle them all over with the seasoning mixture that you didn't reserve in the cereal bowl. Get all sides. Then stick them in the oven and set your timer for 25 minutes (or 20 or 30; timing is not extra-critical here).

4. While the ribs are roasting, stir the broth or beer and the oil into the reserved rub.

5. When the timer goes off, baste the ribs with the broth-oil mixture, turning them over as you do so. Stick them back in the oven and set the timer for another 20 minutes.

6. Repeat for a good 1½ to 2 hours; you want your ribs sizzling brown all over and tender when you pierce them with a fork. Cut into individual ribs to serve.

6 servings. Per serving: 474 calories, 25 g protein, 2 g carbohydrate, 40 g fat, trace fiber

Soy and Sesame Pork Steak

Shoulder steaks are our favorite cut of pork. We've been known to eat them 3 days running!

> **2 tablespoons soy sauce**
> **½ teaspoon dark sesame oil**
> **2 teaspoons Splenda or Sucanat**
> **½ teaspoon chili garlic paste**
> **½ pound pork shoulder steak, about ¼" thick**
> **2 teaspoons coconut oil or olive oil**

1. Mix together the soy sauce, sesame oil, Splenda or Sucanat, and chili garlic paste. Lay the pork steak on a plate with a rim and pour this mixture over it, turning to coat. Let it sit for 15 minutes or so.

2. Give your big skillet a shot of cooking spray and put it over medium-high heat. Melt the coconut oil or olive oil. Now throw in your pork steak. Give it 5 to 7 minutes on each side—you want it browned on the outside and done through but not dried out.

3. Pour any leftover marinade from the plate over the cooked steak in the skillet. Flip the steak once or twice, cooking for another 30 to 60 seconds on each side, then serve.

2 servings. Per serving: 262 calories, 16 g protein, 2 g carbohydrate, 21 g fat, trace fiber

Pork with Lemon-Scallion Topping

Bright, sunny flavor!

> 1 tablespoon olive oil
> 1 pound pork shoulder steaks or thin pork chops
> ¼ cup lemon juice
> 4 teaspoons soy sauce
> 4 teaspoons Splenda or sugar
> 12 scallions, including the crisp greens, thinly sliced
> Salt and ground black pepper to taste

1. Give your big, heavy skillet a shot of cooking spray, then put it over medium heat. Add the oil and slosh it around. When the pan is hot, throw in your pork steaks or pork chops. Let them cook through, turning once; they should be nicely browned on both sides.

2. While the pork is cooking, stir together the lemon juice, soy sauce, and Splenda or sugar.

3. Transfer the steaks to serving plates. Now add the lemon juice mixture and scallions to the skillet and stir around, scraping up any tasty browned bits from the bottom.

4. Let the mixture cook down until it's slightly syrupy. Pour over the pork, scraping the pan to get all of it, season with salt and pepper, and serve.

3 servings. Per serving: 339 calories, 21 g protein, 8 g carbohydrate, 25 g fat, 2 g fiber

Southwestern Pork with Peach Salsa

Boneless pork loin is so lean it can be bland. Not here!

> 2 tablespoons olive oil
> 1½ pounds boneless pork loin, sliced ½" thick
> ¼ cup chicken broth
> 2 teaspoons chili powder
> ½ teaspoon minced garlic
> ¼ teaspoon ground cumin
> 1 tablespoon dry white wine
> 2 tablespoons lime juice
> 1 chipotle chile pepper canned in adobo
> ⅔ cup frozen peach slices
> ⅓ cucumber
> ¼ medium red onion
> ½ jalapeño chile pepper (wear plastic gloves when
>   handling)
> 2 teaspoons rice vinegar
> 1 dash hot-pepper sauce
> Salt to taste

1. In your big, heavy skillet, heat the oil over medium-high heat. Add the pork and brown it lightly on both sides.

2. While that's happening, combine the broth, chili powder, garlic, cumin, wine, and lime juice. Chop the chipotle pepper. When the pork is golden on both sides, pour the broth mixture into the skillet and stir in the chipotle pepper. Turn the heat to medium and let the mixture simmer, uncovered, for 6 to 7 minutes.

3. Meanwhile, put the peach slices, cucumber, onion, jalapeño pepper, vinegar, and hot-pepper sauce in your food processor with the S blade in place and pulse until everything is chopped medium-fine. Add salt and pulse once or twice more.

4. Turn over your pork. Let it simmer for another 5 to 6 minutes. Serve with some of the pan liquid and the peach salsa on top.

4 servings. Per serving: 316 calories, 32 g protein, 13 g carbohydrate, 15 g fat, 2 g fiber

Slow-Cooker Ham Dinner

Everyone loves ham, but it's not the sort of thing you can make on a weeknight. It just takes too darned long. Your slow cooker to the rescue! (This takes a big slow cooker, though.)

>   5 medium turnips
>   2 pounds green cabbage
>   5 pounds ham (half a ham)
>   1 cup chicken broth

1. Peel the turnips and cut them into eighths. Throw them into your slow cooker. Core the cabbage, cut it into chunks, and throw it in too.

2. Now nestle the ham down among all those veggies. It'll take a little doing to fit it down far enough for the lid to go on the slow cooker; you may have to make a hole in the veggies.

3. When your ham is in far enough that you can put the lid on the slow cooker, pour in the broth, slap on the lid, and set the heat to low. Forget about it for 8 hours.

4. When dinnertime rolls around, lift out the ham and put it on a platter. Using a slotted spoon, fish out the veggies and pile them around the ham, and serve. Butter is good on the vegetables, but they'll be flavorful without it.

10 servings. Per serving: 461 calories, 38 g protein, 9 g carbohydrate, 30 g fat, 3 g fiber

Indian Lamb Skillet Supper

This exotic and wonderful dish is a great illustration of how you can use cauliflower "rice" in place of starchy grains.

¾ **pound ground lamb**
½ **large head cauliflower**
½ **medium onion**
2 **cloves garlic, minced**
2 **tablespoons finely chopped fresh mint**
1 **tablespoon finely chopped fresh cilantro**
1 **teaspoon grated fresh ginger**
¾ **teaspoon beef bouillon concentrate**
¾ **teaspoon chicken bouillon concentrate**
½ **teaspoon ground turmeric**
½ **teaspoon ground cumin**
1 **tablespoon lime juice**
1 **teaspoon Splenda or sugar**

1. In a big skillet over medium heat, start the lamb browning.

2. Meanwhile, trim the leaves and the very bottom of the stem from the cauliflower and whack it into chunks. Run it through the shredding blade of your food processor. Put the shredded cauliflower in a microwaveable baking dish with a lid. Add a couple of tablespoons of water, cover, and microwave on high for 6 minutes.

3. Add the onion and garlic to the lamb and continue cooking and crumbling until all the pink is gone from the lamb and the onion is translucent.

4. Pull the cauliflower out of the microwave, uncover immediately to stop the cooking, and drain. Add to the lamb mixture.

5. Stir in the mint, cilantro, ginger, bouillon concentrates, turmeric, and cumin. Stir until everything is well distributed and the bouillon concentrates are dissolved.

6. In a small dish, stir the lime juice and Splenda or sugar together and add to the lamb. Mix together and serve.

3 servings. Per serving: 361 calories, 21 g protein, 9 g carbohydrate, 27 g fat, 3 g fiber

Orange-Rosemary Glazed Lamb Chops

We love lamb chops, but they're pricey. So we also make this recipe with lamb steaks instead. When whole legs of lamb are on sale, we have the nice meat guys cut a chunk off either end for small roasts and slice the rest ¾" thick for steaks. These lamb steaks are lean, meaty, and wonderful—and cheaper than lamb chops!

> 1½ pounds lamb chops or lamb leg steaks, in 4 portions
> 2 tablespoons spicy brown mustard, divided
> 1 tablespoon olive oil
> 2 tablespoons low-sugar orange preserves
> ¼ cup dry white wine
> ½ teaspoon ground rosemary
> 1 teaspoon lemon juice
> ½ teaspoon Splenda or sugar

1. Give your big, heavy skillet a shot of cooking spray and put it over medium heat.

2. While the pan is heating, spread each side of the chops or steaks with ½ teaspoon of the mustard, using 4 teaspoons mustard total.

3. Add the oil to the pan and throw in your chops or steaks. While they are browning, mix together the rest of the mustard, the orange preserves, wine, rosemary, lemon juice, and Splenda.

4. Flip the lamb chops or steaks. Cook until good and brown on the outside but pink in the middle. Transfer to serving plates.

5. Pour the preserves mixture into the skillet and mix it around, scraping up any brown crusty bits in the skillet. Let it cook down until it's syrupy, pour it over the meat, and serve.

4 servings. Per serving: 475 calories, 23 g protein, 4 g carbohydrate, 40 g fat, trace fiber

Slow-Cooker Lamb Shanks

Tough, cheap, flavorful lamb shanks are perfect for slow cooking. They come out fork-tender and utterly delicious. With Fauxtatoes (page 223), they're scrumptious.

1 tablespoon olive oil
2 pounds lamb shanks (2 good-size shanks, but be sure they'll fit into your slow cooker!)
2 medium onions, sliced
8 ounces sliced mushrooms
¼ cup dry white wine
¼ cup tomato sauce
½ teaspoon paprika
½ teaspoon ground ginger
½ teaspoon beef bouillon concentrate
½ teaspoon ground black pepper
½ cup chicken broth
Guar or xanthan

1. Coat your big, heavy skillet with cooking spray and put it over medium-high heat. Add the oil and throw in the lamb shanks. You're searing them. You want to get them good and brown all over their surface.

2. While the lamb shanks are searing, haul out your slow cooker and throw in the onions and mushrooms. Stir together everything else but the guar or xanthan (be sure the bouillon is dissolved).

3. When the shanks are nicely browned, put them on top of the veggies in the slow cooker. Pour the sauce over everything, cover the pot, set it on low, and let it cook for 8 to 10 hours.

4. When it's time to serve, pull out the lamb shanks and put them on a platter. Use your guar or xanthan shaker to thicken up the sauce just a tad—to about the texture of cream.

5. Carve each shank into 2 portions of meat and serve with Fauxtatoes, piling the onions and mushrooms over everything and pouring the sauce over it all.

4 servings. Per serving: 452 calories, 36 g protein, 9 g carbohydrate, 28 g fat, 2 g fiber (Analysis does not include Fauxtatoes.)

Savory Greek Lamb Shanks and Lima Beans

The robust flavorings of this dish are decidedly Greek, thanks to the marinated olives, oregano, cinnamon, and garlic. Instead of the traditional roasted potatoes, this lamb is paired with super-garlicky lima beans, creating a robust meal that would satisfy Zorba.

> 1 tablespoon extra virgin olive oil
> 4 lamb shanks (about 1 pound each), trimmed of excess fat
> Salt and ground black pepper to taste
> 1 medium onion, sliced (2 cups)
> ½ teaspoon dried oregano
> 2 teaspoons ground cinnamon
> 5 cloves garlic, minced, divided
> ½ cup red wine or chicken stock
> 1 can (15 ounces) tomatoes, drained
> Peel of ½ small lemon
> ½ cup marinated black or green olives
> 1 package (10 ounces) frozen baby lima beans
> 1 tablespoon chopped parsley

1. Heat the oil in a deep skillet or baking dish with a tight-fitting lid. Add the lamb shanks and cook for about 10 minutes over medium-high heat, browning on all sides and seasoning with salt and pepper. Transfer the meat to a platter.

2. Pour off all but 2 tablespoons of fat from the skillet. Add the onion and cook over medium heat for about 10 minutes, stirring occasionally, until soft and golden. Stir in the oregano, the cinnamon, and 2 cloves of the garlic and cook for another minute.

3. Add the wine or stock, tomatoes, and lemon peel and stir to mix. Return the lamb to the skillet, turning it in the sauce to coat it on all sides. Cover and cook on low heat for 30 minutes.

4. Turn over the lamb shanks, add the olives and the remaining 3 cloves of garlic, and cover the skillet. Cook for another 30 minutes.

5. Add the lima beans, making sure they are completely covered with sauce, adding wine if necessary. Continue cooking the lamb

mixture until the meat is very tender and nearly falling off the bone, about 1 hour.

6. Place a lamb shank on each dinner plate, along with a generous amount of the cooking sauce and beans. Sprinkle with the parsley. For a feast, add a Greek salad topped with feta cheese.

4 servings. Per serving: 484 calories, 48 g protein, 30 g carbohydrate, 17 g fat, 9 g fiber

23

Fish and Seafood

Fish has long been considered the healthiest of animal foods. It's true that fish is a great source of protein and often of good fats as well. It has the added advantage of cooking quickly.

But we've learned that some of what made fish look so healthy compared with red meat was that, until recently, most of it was wild caught, not farmed. Turns out that feeding grains and beans to fish causes the same kinds of shifts in fatty acid profiles that we see in grain-fed beef. Doesn't make fish bad for you—but it does mean that wild-caught fish are worth paying extra for if your budget will stretch.

Seafood Favorites

Seafood is carb free, high in protein, and low in saturated fat. It's best prepared in ways that bring out its distinct, subtle flavors. You can cook it in a skillet or broil, grill, bake, or poach it—just don't overcook it. Enhance it with flavored butters, oils, sauces, salsas, and vinaigrettes—the possibilities are endless. Here are some classic ways to enjoy fish, followed by our own low-glycemic-load recipes.

- **Sole meunière:** In this simple French preparation of sole, fillets of fish are dredged in flour, cooked in butter and olive oil, and served with lemon slices and parsley. You can substitute any mild fish fillet.
- **Fish tacos:** After marinating and grilling swordfish, halibut, or any other firm fish, you can slice it and serve it with shredded lettuce and your favorite salsa, wrapped in a low-carb tortilla.
- **Seafood gumbo:** This thick stew originated in Louisiana and is traditionally made with shrimp, scallops, lobster, and crab combined with sausage and bell peppers, onions, tomatoes, and, most important, okra.

Seared Fish with Ginger-Lime Cucumber Dipping Sauce

This is nothing short of amazing, and it's so quick and easy. The cucumber shreds hold the sauce on the fish and add a cool note of their own. You have to try this!

Ginger-Lime Dipping Sauce
2 tablespoons grated fresh ginger
2 cloves garlic, crushed
2 tablespoons Splenda or sugar
Juice of ½ lime
2 tablespoons water
2 tablespoons fish sauce (nuoc mam or nam pla)
½ teaspoon chili garlic paste, or to taste

Fish
½ cucumber
1 tablespoon coconut oil or peanut oil
Salt and ground black pepper to taste
3 fish fillets—sea bass, red snapper, orange roughy, sole, flounder, or tilapia (about 18 ounces)

1. First make your dipping sauce, which is extremely easy—just mix together the ginger, garlic, Splenda or sugar, lime juice, water, fish sauce, and chili garlic paste.

2. To make the fish, use the tip of a spoon to scrape the seeds out of the cucumber half. Run the cucumber flesh through the shredding disk of your food processor or shred it on a box grater. Either way, try to get the longest strands you can. (In your food processor, this means laying chunks of cucumber down in the feed tube so they get shredded the long way, instead of across.)Gather up your shredded cuke and plunk it into the bowl of dipping sauce.

3. Give your big, heavy skillet a shot of cooking spray and put it over medium-high heat. Let it get hot, then add the oil and slosh it around to coat the skillet.

4. Salt and pepper the fillets on both sides and throw them into the fat. Give them about 5 minutes per side—you want them done through but not dry, and nicely browned on both sides. Transfer to serving plates.

5. Using a fork, fish the cucumber strands out of the dipping sauce and divide them equally among the fillets, piling them on top. Drizzle a little more of the sauce from the dish over each fillet and serve immediately.

3 servings. Per serving: 222 calories, 31 g protein, 7 g carbohydrate, 7 g fat, 1 g fiber

Baked Perch in Roasted Red Bell Pepper–Sun-Dried Tomato Sauce

This quick and easy recipe drew raves from dinner party company.

>6 ocean perch fillets (about 1½ pounds)
>2 tablespoons lemon juice
>Salt and ground black pepper to taste
>1 cup roasted red bell peppers jarred in water, drained
>1 cup oil-packed sun-dried tomatoes, drained
>½ cup dry white wine
>1 small onion, quartered
>2 cloves garlic, chopped
>1 teaspoon Creole seasoning (Tony Chachere's is good)

1. Preheat the oven to 350°F.

2. Spray a shallow enamel, glass, or stainless steel baking dish with cooking spray. Lay the perch fillets skin side down in the prepared baking dish. Sprinkle with the lemon juice and salt and pepper. Set aside.

3. Put the roasted bell peppers, sun-dried tomatoes, wine, onion, garlic, and Creole seasoning in your food processor with the S blade in place and pulse until the bell peppers, tomatoes, and onion are chopped medium-fine. Spoon the resulting sauce evenly over the fish fillets.

4. Bake uncovered for 20 to 25 minutes, transfer to plates, and serve.

6 servings. Per serving: 175 calories, 23 g protein, 8 g carbohydrate, 5 g fat, 2 g fiber

Easy and Elegant Salmon Packets

Exactly what the name says—and no pan to wash!

>4 salmon fillets (about 1 pound)
>Salt and ground black pepper to taste
>8 thin slices lemon
>4 sprigs fresh dill
>2 tablespoons dry vermouth

1. Preheat the oven to 375°F.

2. Tear off 4 roughly 12" squares of foil. Lay a salmon fillet in the middle of each. Salt and pepper them.

3. Now cover each fillet with 2 thin lemon slices and top with a sprig of dill. Sprinkle ½ tablespoon vermouth over each.

4. Fold up the sides of the foil and roll down. Then roll up the ends. Place the packets in a pan, in case of leaks, and bake for 20 to 25 minutes. Serve in the foil, letting diners open their own packets.

4 servings. Per serving: 147 calories, 23 g protein, 3 g carbohydrate, 4 g fat, trace fiber

Bass with Sour Cream–Roasted Red Bell Pepper Sauce

With this fish and a salad of spinach or mixed baby greens in a simple vinaigrette, you've got a dinner any restaurant would be proud of—in less than a half hour, tops!

Salt and ground black pepper to taste
4 sea bass fillets (about 1½ pounds)
2 tablespoons lemon juice
½ teaspoon dried thyme
½ cup light sour cream
1 teaspoon Dijon or spicy brown mustard
1 teaspoon ketchup
2 tablespoons finely chopped roasted red bell peppers jarred in water
2 scallions, including the crisp greens, minced

1. Preheat the oven to 400°F. Spray a baking dish that has a lid with cooking spray. (If you don't have a covered baking dish that fits your fillets, you can use a glass baking pan and cover it tightly with foil.)

2. Lightly salt and pepper your bass fillets and lay them in the baking dish. Sprinkle the lemon juice and thyme over them. Cover the baking dish and place it in the oven. Bake for 8 to 10 minutes.

3. While the fish is baking, stir together the sour cream, mustard, ketchup, roasted red bell pepper, and one of the minced scallions.

4. Uncover the fish. Spread the sour cream mixture evenly over the fillets and return them to the oven. Bake for 2 to 3 minutes longer.

5. Serve the bass with the second minced scallion scattered over it for garnish.

4 servings. Per serving: 214 calories, 33 g protein, 4 g carbohydrate, 7 g fat, 1 g fiber

Caramelized Shrimp

This is Vietnamese in inspiration.

>2 tablespoons peanut oil or coconut oil
>1 pound large E-Z peel shrimp
>1½ tablespoons Sucanat, or 1½ tablespoons Splenda plus
> ⅛ teaspoon blackstrap molasses (or the darkest
> available)
>1 clove garlic, crushed
>1 shallot, finely chopped
>¼ cup water
>1 tablespoon fish sauce (nuoc mam or nam pla)
>¼ teaspoon salt
>¼ cup finely chopped fresh cilantro

1. Have everything prepped and ready to go before you start cooking.

2. Put your biggest skillet over medium heat and add the oil. When it's hot, throw in the shrimp. Sprinkle the Sucanat or Splenda and molasses over them and stir-fry for 1 minute.

3. Add the garlic and shallot and stir-fry for another minute. Now add the water, fish sauce, and salt. Turn the heat down to medium-low and let the shrimp cook for another minute or two, until the pan is just about dry and the shrimp are cooked through.

4. Divide the shrimp among 3 plates, top each with a table-spoon of chopped cilantro, and serve.

3 servings. Per serving: 240 calories, 25 g protein, 9 g carbohydrate, 11 g fat, trace fiber

Shrimp with Garlic, Chile, and Herbs

This scrumptious shrimp dish needs no sales pitch with all its lively seasonings. Low-glycemic-load eating is a pleasure with dishes like this one. You can use fresh or frozen shrimp sold in most supermarkets.

> 1 medium tomato, chopped
> 1 hot chile pepper, such as a serrano pepper, chopped (wear plastic gloves when handling)
> 2 tablespoons extra virgin olive oil, divided
> ½ cup fresh cilantro
> 2 tablespoons fresh mint leaves
> 1 pound shrimp, peeled and deveined, with tails left on
> 4 cloves garlic, minced
> ½ teaspoon salt

1. In a large skillet, cook the tomato and chile pepper in 1 tablespoon of the oil over medium heat until somewhat softened, about 5 minutes.

2. Put the cilantro and mint in a food processor fitted with a metal blade, and add the tomato and chile pepper. Process to the consistency of a sauce.

3. Heat the remaining 1 tablespoon of oil in the skillet over medium heat. Add the shrimp. Cook, stirring occasionally, for 2 minutes. Add the garlic and salt; stir and cook for 2 more minutes, until the shrimp are nearly opaque.

4. Reduce the heat to low and pour in the tomato mixture. Stir to combine. Cook until the shrimp are opaque but still tender, about 5 minutes. Serve immediately. Tasty accompaniments are black beans cooked with a clove of garlic; vinaigrette salad made with avocado, tomato, and red bell pepper; and Mexican beer.

4 servings. Per serving: 191 calories, 25 g protein, 4 g carbohydrate, 8 g fat, 1 g fiber

Asian Steamed Scallops

We made this in little heatproof ramekins, but if you have nice decorative scallop shells, use them instead—though they'll be harder to fit into your steamer! (If you don't own a steamer, bamboo ones are available cheaply at Asian markets and import stores.) As it is, you may need to do this in two batches. This would also make a good appetizer for eight—one scallop per serving instead of two.

> 8 very large scallops (about 1 pound)
> Salt and ground black pepper to taste
> 8 thin slices fresh ginger, plus 2 tablespoons grated
> 6 scallions
> 4 cloves garlic
> ½ teaspoon chili paste
> ¼ cup soy sauce
> 4 teaspoons dark sesame oil
> 2 teaspoons water
> 1½ teaspoons Splenda

1. Start water heating in a pot that will fit your steamer.
2. Put 2 scallops each into 4 small heatproof dishes. Salt and pepper them lightly.
3. Use a sharp knife to cut the ginger slices into skinny little strips, the thinner the better. Trim the roots and any wilted parts of the green tops off the scallions. Now separate the crisp green parts from the white parts. Cut the green parts lengthwise into long, skinny strips. Whack the white parts into 2 or 3 pieces each.
4. Whack the garlic cloves with the flat side of your knife to loosen the skin. Pick the skin off and then finely mince 1 clove.
5. Scatter the skinny strips of ginger and scallion greens, plus the minced garlic, over the scallops, dividing them equally.
6. By now your water should be boiling. Put the dishes in your steamer and put the steamer over the boiling water. Cover and steam for 10 to 12 minutes, until the scallops are opaque and have firmed up.

(continued)

7. While that's happening, put the white parts of the scallions and the remaining cloves of garlic into your food processor with the S blade in place. Add the chili paste, soy sauce, sesame oil, water, Splenda, and grated ginger, and whirl until the garlic and scallion are finely minced. This is your sauce.

8. When the scallops are done, put each dish on a small plate, with a little puddle of the sauce for dipping, and serve.

4 servings. Per serving: 223 calories, 27 g protein, 11 g carbohydrate, 7 g fat, 1 g fiber

Grilled Halibut with Lemon-Herb Splash

If grilling is not your thing, you can pan-sear or bake the fish. Sea bass is a delicious alternative to the halibut. The lemon-herb splash also makes a great marinade for grilled prawns or sea scallops. (This recipe is from *Dishing with Kathy Casey*.)

6 tablespoons extra virgin olive oil
2 tablespoons fresh lemon juice
2 teaspoons lemon peel
1½ teaspoons finely chopped fresh rosemary
1½ teaspoons finely chopped fresh basil
1 tablespoon finely chopped parsley
⅛ teaspoon dried red-pepper flakes
½ teaspoon minced garlic
¼ teaspoon salt
4 halibut steaks or fillets (1½ pounds)
Oil as needed
Salt and ground black pepper to taste

1. To make the lemon-herb splash, mix together the olive oil, lemon juice, lemon peel, rosemary, basil, parsley, red-pepper flakes, garlic, and salt. Refrigerate until needed.

2. Preheat the grill. Lightly rub the fish on each side with a little oil and season with salt and pepper as desired.

3. Grill the fish for 2 to 3 minutes per side, depending on its thickness. The fish should be nicely grill-marked and cooked through but still juicy.

4. Place the fish on plates and pour 1 tablespoon or more of the lemon-herb splash over each piece of fish. Pass the remaining splash on the side.

4 servings. Per serving: 420 calories, 46 g protein, 1 g carbohydrate, 25 g fat, trace fiber

Note: To add a light smoky flavor, soak a few apple, mesquite, or pecan wood chips (depending on where you live) in water. Throw them on the coals just before placing the fish on the grill.

Deviled Catfish

Catfish is usually dredged in cornmeal and deep-fried in questionable fat—tasty, but not exactly great for you. Mixing cornmeal and almond meal keeps the flavor and the crunch while lowering the glycemic load.

¼ cup whole grain cornmeal
½ cup almond meal
1 teaspoon crab-boil seasoning
¼ cup brown mustard
1½ tablespoons hot-pepper sauce
1 tablespoon coconut oil
1 tablespoon olive oil
1 pound catfish nuggets or fillets

1. On a plate, mix together the cornmeal, almond meal, and crab-boil seasoning. In a dish, mix together the mustard and hot-pepper sauce.

2. Give your big, heavy skillet a squirt of cooking spray and put it over medium-high heat. Add the oils and start them heating; meal slosh them together as the coconut oil melts.

3. Dip the catfish in the mustard–hot-pepper sauce mixture, using a fork to turn until coated well. Then drop into the cornmeal–almond-meal mixture, again turning to coat. As they're coated, drop each nugget or fillet in the hot fat and fry until crispy all over, turning them over to brown. Serve hot.

4 servings. Per serving: 280 calories, 27 g protein, 12 g carbohydrate, 15 g fat, 1 g fiber

Creamed Tuna with Noodles

Remember that tuna-noodle casserole your mom used to make with the canned cream of mushroom soup and the peas? The one that was so humble, homey, comfy—and yummy? This is a dead ringer—but with the starchy stuff cut out.

> 1 tablespoon butter
> ½ medium onion, chopped
> 2 cups chopped mushrooms
> 1 cup frozen peas
> 1 can (12 ounces) tuna packed in water, drained
> 1½ cups half-and-half
> 1½ teaspoons Worcestershire sauce
> 1 teaspoon beef bouillon concentrate
> 16 ounces tofu shirataki noodles (fettuccine width)
> Salt and ground black pepper to taste

1. In a big saucepan over medium-low heat, melt the butter and start cooking the onion and mushrooms, stirring frequently.

2. While that's happening, put the still-frozen peas in a microwaveable bowl. Add a tablespoon or so of water, cover with a plate or saucer, and microwave on high for 4 minutes.

3. When the mushrooms have softened and changed color and the onion is translucent, drain the peas and dump them into the pan. Add the tuna too. Pour in the half-and-half and stir in the Worcestershire and bouillon concentrate. Let the whole thing come to a simmer, stirring now and then. When the mixture is at a simmer, adjust the heat to keep it there (instead of boiling hard) and let it simmer for 8 to 10 minutes.

4. Meanwhile, snip open the shirataki packets and drain them. When the 8 to 10 minutes is up, dump in the noodles and stir them in. Add salt and pepper to taste, and serve.

4 servings. Per serving: 303 calories, 31 g protein, 12 g carbohydrate, 14 g fat, 2 g fiber

Note: Buy chunk light tuna rather than the more expensive white—i.e., albacore—tuna. Chunk light has far less mercury.

Hot Tuna Wraps

We tried heating these on my electric tabletop grill, but the filling squeezed out all over the place! So heat them in the oven.

1 can (6 ounces) tuna packed in water, drained
2 ounces Swiss cheese, finely chopped
2 ounces sharp Cheddar cheese, finely chopped
3 hard-cooked eggs, peeled and chopped
¼ medium green bell pepper, finely chopped
¼ medium onion, finely chopped
2 tablespoons chopped pimiento-stuffed green olives
2 tablespoons sweet pickle relish
¼ cup light mayonnaise
5 large low-carb tortillas

1. Preheat the oven to 350°F.
2. Drain the tuna and place it in a mixing bowl. Flake it thoroughly with a fork. Add the cheeses, eggs, bell pepper, onion, olives, relish, and mayonnaise and mix well.
3. Lay a large tortilla on a plate and put 3 rounded tablespoons of the tuna mixture on it. Fold up the bottom, then fold in the sides and roll. Place the filled tortillas seam side down on a baking sheet and bake for 20 minutes. Serve hot.

5 servings. Per serving: 298 calories, 19 g protein, 24 g carbohydrate, 16 g fat, 14 g fiber

Salmon with Mushrooms and Crème Fraîche

Salmon steaks and fillets can be dry, but there's little chance of that with this recipe. The fish is gently cooked on low heat and served with a creamy sauce that moistens every last mouthful of this delectable dish. And wait until you taste the combination of salmon and fragrant mushrooms, a surprisingly compatible pairing of flavors.

> **3 tablespoons unrefined safflower oil**
> **3 cloves garlic, minced**
> **8 ounces mixed fresh mushrooms such as cremini, oyster, shiitake, and porcini**
> **4 salmon fillets or steaks, about ¾" thick (1 pound)**
> **Salt to taste**
> **½ cup crème fraîche (see note)**
> **1 teaspoon lemon juice**
> **1 tablespoon finely chopped parsley**
> **Salt and ground black pepper to taste**

1. In a large skillet over medium heat, warm the oil. Add the garlic and cook for 1 minute, taking care that the garlic doesn't brown. Add the mushrooms and cook, stirring frequently, for 2 minutes.

2. Lay the salmon (skin side down if using fillets) on the bed of mushrooms in the skillet. Season the fish and vegetables with salt. Cover the skillet, lower the heat, and cook until the flesh of the fish is no longer opaque but is still moist, about 6 minutes. Using a slotted spatula, transfer the fish and mushrooms to dinner plates.

3. Add the crème fraîche to the liquid remaining in the skillet. If the sauce is scant or too thick, add 1 or 2 tablespoons water. Stir in the lemon juice and season to taste. Add the parsley, stir, and spoon the sauce over the fish.

4 servings. Per serving: 342 calories, 31 g protein, 6 g carbohydrate, 21 g fat, 1 g fiber

Note: A French specialty, crème fraîche has a slightly tangy, nutty flavor and velvety, rich texture. It can be boiled without curdling, making it an ideal addition to sauces such as this one.

Weeknight Fish Stew

This concoction of seafood and vegetables tastes like a complicated dish but goes together quickly—especially if you buy fish with all the bones removed and deveined shrimp. Of course, you can make the stew more elaborate by adding shellfish and sausage, but this version delivers lots of flavor as it is. Parsnips add sweetness.

> 2 tablespoons extra virgin olive oil
> 1 cup chopped onion
> 2 parsnips, peeled and cut into 1" chunks
> 2 carrots, peeled and cut into 1" chunks
> 1 can (15 ounces) no-salt-added chicken broth
> 1 can (15 ounces) stewed tomatoes
> Hot-pepper sauce to taste
> 2 cloves garlic, minced
> 1¼ pounds assorted fish, such as cod, halibut, and red
>   snapper, skin and bones removed
> 12 large deveined shrimp, shells removed
> ¼ pound spinach, thoroughly washed and coarsely
>   chopped
> Salt and ground black pepper to taste

1. Heat the oil over medium-high heat in a large saucepan with a lid. Add the onion and cook, stirring frequently, until it softens and becomes translucent, about 7 minutes.

2. Add the parsnips, carrots, broth, and tomatoes. Cover and cook on medium-high heat until the vegetables are just tender, about 20 minutes.

3. Stir in the hot-pepper sauce and garlic. Add the fish, submerging it in the tomato sauce as much as possible. Cook on medium heat for 5 to 10 minutes until the fish is opaque and tender.

4. Add the shrimp and cook for 2 minutes. Immediately add the spinach, cover the pot, and cook until the spinach wilts, 2 to 3 minutes. At this point, the shrimp should be pink all over but still tender. Season with salt and pepper. Serve with a green salad.

4 servings. Per serving: 429 calories, 49 g protein, 35 g carbohydrate, 10 g fat, 9 g fiber

24

Desserts

Y ou can satisfy your sweet tooth and still keep your glycemic load down. The trick is to use desserts and sweets
to stimulate your tastebuds, not to fill up on. This is
where the difference between glycemic index and glycemic load
becomes crucial. You can enjoy foods with high glycemic
indexes, as long as you don't eat enough to raise your glycemic
load. If the sugar isn't diluted with starch, as it is in cookies,
cakes, and pastries, a typical-size serving after a meal shouldn't
cause a glucose shock.

What Can You Have?

Be careful, though; sweets are so pleasing to the palate that you
might get carried away, even when you're not hungry. So enjoy
these dessert options and recipes in moderation.

- **Chocolate:** From the finest dark chocolate truffle to the
  ubiquitous chocolate chip, chocolate is your friend as long
  as you use it to satisfy your sweet tooth, not your hunger. The
  glycemic load of dark or semisweet chocolate is lower than
  that of milk chocolate. I keep Ghirardelli double-chocolate,
  dark chocolate chips in the freezer and grab some when I

Dr. Rob Says:
How Sugar Can Be Your Friend

You can't taste starch. Enzymes in your saliva break down a tiny fraction of the starch you eat into sugar, which you can taste, but otherwise it's flavorless. However, as soon as it hits your stomach, it turns to sugar. Scientists infused sugar through tubes inserted directly into people's stomachs and compared their eating behaviors with those of people fed sugar orally. The sugar that people could taste suppressed appetite more than sugar they couldn't taste.

People tend to consume more sugar when it is delivered to their bloodstream in the form of starch than they do when it is in the form of table sugar or candy. A good trick for ridding yourself of the urge to eat starch is to finish your meal and have a couple of pieces of candy. You might find that you're more satisfied and end up consuming less sugar.

A pile of sugar would raise your blood sugar as much as a similar-size pile of bread, potatoes, or rice. The difference is the serving size. You would never eat as much sugar in one sitting as you would the starch. It's too sweet. The same is true for other candy as long as you can taste all the sugar in it. A few bits of chocolate after dinner can make life enjoyable if you have a sweet tooth and would contribute little to glycemic load.

have a craving for something sweet. Just remember the rules: Eat them after a meal, and don't eat more than you can wrap the fingers of one hand around.

- **Chocolate-covered nuts:** Nuts are carb free, and there isn't enough sugar in a coating of chocolate to make much of an impact, as long as this candy is consumed in moderation.

- **Peanut brittle, peppermint candy, and jelly beans:** These nonstarchy candies are fine as long as you consume them only after a meal and don't eat more than you can wrap your fingers around.
- **Sugar-free ice cream:** The high sugar content of most ice creams results in unacceptable glycemic loads. However, some companies are making no-sugar-added ice creams, which have low glycemic loads. Be careful not to confuse these with low-fat ice creams, which are usually very high in sugar.

For the following recipes, we've walked the middle path where sugar is concerned. We've used some Sucanat and some Splenda, while concentrating on keeping total carb load low.

Cookie Mix

With this mix in the refrigerator, you're never more than 20 minutes from fresh-baked cookies. Feel free to substitute Splenda for up to two-thirds of the Sucanat in this recipe. If you do, subtract 2 grams of carbohydrate from each cookie you make from the mix.

> 1½ pounds (6 sticks) butter
> 3 cups Sucanat
> 1½ cups oat bran
> 1½ cups wheat germ
> 3 cups almond meal
> 3 cups vanilla whey protein powder
> 3 cups powdered milk (the instant skim milk at your
>   grocery store will do fine)
> ¾ cup sesame seeds (see note)
> 1 tablespoon salt
> 3 tablespoons baking powder

Put everything in your food processor with the S blade in place and pulse until the butter is cut in and dispersed evenly. Store in an airtight container in the fridge or freezer.

Makes a gallon of mix, which will make about 192 cookies. Per cookie: 81 calories, 4 g protein, 6 g carbohydrate, 5 g fat, 1 g fiber

Note: Buy sesame seeds in bulk at a health food store; they'll be far cheaper than if you buy them in a little bottle off the spice rack. If your health food store offers them, choose unhulled sesame seeds instead of the familiar hulled variety—they're higher in minerals and fiber.

Here are some ways to use your cookie mix. The directions for all of the following recipes are the same: Preheat the oven to 350°F. Spray a baking sheet with cooking spray. Use your electric mixer to combine everything well. Drop by rounded tablespoonfuls onto the baking sheet. Bake for 12 to 15 minutes, then cool on a rack.

Almond Cookies from Mix

2 cups Cookie Mix (page 316)
1 egg
¾ cup almond butter
1 teaspoon vanilla extract
½ teaspoon almond extract

2 dozen cookies. Per cookie: 134 calories, 5 g protein, 8 g carbohydrate, 10 g fat, 1 g fiber

Peanut Butter Cookies from Mix

2 cups Cookie Mix (page 316)
1 egg
¾ cup natural peanut butter
1 teaspoon vanilla extract

2 dozen cookies. Per cookie: 131 calories, 6 g protein, 8 g carbohydrate, 9 g fat, 1 g fiber

Sesame Cookies from Mix

2 cups Cookie Mix (page 316)
1 egg
¾ cup tahini (sesame butter)
1 teaspoon vanilla extract

2 dozen cookies. Per cookie: 129 calories, 6 g protein, 8 g carbohydrate, 9 g fat, 1 g fiber

Spice Cookies from Mix

2 cups Cookie Mix (page 316)
1 egg
1 teaspoon ground cinnamon
Pinch of ground cloves
Pinch of ground nutmeg
1 teaspoon vanilla extract

16 cookies. Per cookie: 127 calories, 6 g protein, 9 g carbohydrate, 8 g fat, 1 g fiber

Chocolate Chip Cookies from Mix

2 cups Cookie Mix (page 316)
1 egg
1 teaspoon vanilla extract
¾ cup chocolate chips

2 dozen cookies. Per cookie: 118 calories, 5 g protein, 10 g carbohydrate, 7 g fat, 1 g fiber

"*Graham*" *Crust*

Here's what you use instead of a graham cracker crumb crust.

> 2 cups All-Bran, All-Bran Extra Fiber,
>   or Fiber One cereal
> ½ cup raw wheat germ
> ¼ cup Splenda
> 4 tablespoons butter, melted
> 3 tablespoons water

1. Preheat the oven to 350°F. Spray a pie plate with cooking spray. (You can use a 9" or a 10" pie plate; with the bigger one you'll just get a thinner crust or perhaps not build it up as high on the sides.)

2. Put the All-Bran into your food processor (with the S blade in place) and run until it's finely ground. Don't stop too soon; we did the first time, and while my crust tasted good, the texture left something to be desired.

3. Add the wheat germ and Splenda and pulse to mix them in. Add the butter and pulse to mix it in.

4. When the butter is distributed evenly, add the water a tablespoon at a time, pulsing to mix in each addition thoroughly before you add the next.

5. Turn the mixture into your prepared pie plate and press firmly on the bottom and up the sides. Bake for 13 to 15 minutes. Cool before filling.

12 servings. Per serving: 80 calories, 2 g protein, 11 g carbohydrate, 5 g fat, 4 g fiber

Lemon-Vanilla Cheesecake

Light, creamy, and lemony. You could top this with fruit if you liked, but it's awfully good as is. Makes a terrific breakfast too.

24 ounces creamed cottage cheese
½ cup plain yogurt
2 eggs
¼ cup vanilla whey protein powder
1 lemon
⅔ cup Splenda
¼ teaspoon salt
1 "Graham" Crust (page 319), made in a 10" pie plate, baked and ready to go

1. Preheat the oven to 325°F.

2. You can make this in your food processor with the S blade or in your blender, though I think a food processor works a little better. Either way, process or blend the cottage cheese until it's absolutely smooth.

3. Add the yogurt, eggs, whey protein powder, lemon, Splenda, and salt and process until everything is very well blended. Pour into your crust. Place in the oven and place another pan with an inch of water in it on the rack below the cheesecake. Bake for 55 to 60 minutes, then remove from the oven and let cool.

4. Chill for several hours. Serve by itself or with fruit.

12 servings. Per serving: 180 calories, 14 g protein, 15 g carbohydrate, 9 g fat, 4 g fiber

Applesauce Spice Cake

Wonderful with a cup of tea or coffee. This makes a nice breakfast.

1½ cups hulled pumpkin seeds (pepitas)
1½ cups vanilla whey protein powder
2 teaspoons baking powder
1 teaspoon baking soda
½ teaspoon salt
2 teaspoons ground ginger
1½ teaspoons ground cinnamon
½ teaspoon ground cloves
1½ cups Splenda, Sucanat, or a combination
2 cups unsweetened applesauce
3 eggs
⅓ cup coconut oil, melted
1 tablespoon blackstrap molasses

1. Preheat the oven to 350°F. Spray a nonstick Bundt pan with cooking spray.

2. Place the pumpkin seeds in your food processor with the S blade in place and grind them to a fine meal. Take a tablespoon or two and sprinkle them over the Bundt pan to "flour" it. Measure the rest; you want 1½ cups pumpkin seed meal. Put it in a mixing bowl.

3. Add the whey protein powder, baking powder, baking soda, salt, ginger, cinnamon, cloves, and Splenda and/or Sucanat. Using a whisk, stir the dry ingredients together until they're distributed evenly.

4. In another bowl, combine the applesauce, eggs, coconut oil, and molasses and whisk them together.

5. Now add the wet ingredients to the dry, using a rubber scraper to make sure you get all the applesauce mixture. Whisk the wet and dry ingredients together, mixing just until you're sure there are no pockets of dry stuff left. Pour the batter into the prepared Bundt pan, again making sure you scrape it all out of the bowl.

6. Bake for 50 to 60 minutes, or until a wooden pick inserted midway between the walls of the cake pan comes out clean. Turn out onto a rack to cool. Tastes great plain, or with a dab of whipped cream.

18 servings. Per serving: 167 calories, 16 g protein, 11 g carbohydrate, 7 g fat, 2 g fiber

Old-Fashioned Apple Bars

These taste like something your great-grandma would have made.

½ cup rolled oats
¼ cup wheat germ
¼ cup flaxseed meal
½ cup almond meal
½ cup vanilla whey protein powder
½ teaspoon salt
½ teaspoon ground cinnamon
8 tablespoons (1 stick) butter
2 smallish Granny Smith or other juicy, tart apples
⅓ cup Splenda
2 tablespoons Sucanat

1. Preheat the oven to 350°F. Spray an 8" × 8" baking dish with cooking spray.
2. Combine the oats, wheat germ, flaxseed meal, almond meal, whey protein powder, salt, and cinnamon in your food processor (with the S blade in place) and pulse quickly to mix. Then add the butter, cut into a few chunks. Pulse until the butter is cut in.
3. Place half of this mixture in the baking dish and press it into an even layer. Put the rest of the grain mixture into a bowl for the time being. Put the food processor bowl back on the base and put the S blade back in.
4. Quarter the apples and cut out the cores and stems. Throw the quarters into the food processor and pulse until they're chopped medium-fine.
5. Layer the apples over the grain mixture in the pan. Sprinkle the Splenda and Sucanat evenly over them. Then crumble the remaining grain mixture over the apples.
6. Bake for 35 minutes; cool a bit before cutting.

9 servings. Per serving: 260 calories, 16 g protein, 17 g carbohydrate, 15 g fat, 4 g fiber

Yummy Apple-Walnut Cake-Pie Thing

Is it a pie? Is it a cake? Who cares? It's irresistible.

¼ cup Sucanat
¾ cup Splenda
¼ cup almond meal
¼ cup vanilla whey protein powder
1 teaspoon baking powder
⅛ teaspoon salt
1 egg
½ teaspoon vanilla extract
2 medium apples, peeled, cored, and chopped
½ cup chopped walnuts

1. Preheat the oven to 350°F. Coat a 9" pie plate with cooking spray.

2. In a wide and shallow mixing bowl, combine the Sucanat, Splenda, almond meal, whey protein powder, baking powder, and salt. Stir together to distribute evenly.

3. Beat the egg with the vanilla extract, then pour it into the dry ingredients. Stir until everything is evenly moist—the mixture will be thick and sticky. Stir in the apples and walnuts.

4. Spread the mixture in your prepared pie plate and bake for 30 minutes.

8 servings. Per serving: 161 calories, 9 g protein, 17 g carbohydrate, 7 g fat, 2 g fiber

Lemon-Scented Macaroons

The richness of coconut marries well with the tartness of citrus in these macaroons. The cookies go together and bake in a jiffy to give you the ideal garnish for a mixed-fruit dessert of sliced fresh oranges and banana.

> 2 egg whites
> 1 teaspoon vanilla extract
> Peel of 1 lemon, preferably organic
> 2½ cups coconut
> ¾ cup sugar
> Pinch of salt

1. Preheat the oven to 350°F. Cover a baking sheet with parchment paper.

2. Briefly beat the egg whites, vanilla, and lemon peel in a large bowl with a fork. Add the coconut, sugar, and salt. Combine the ingredients, using a wooden spoon or your hands.

3. Manually make small piles of the mixture, each about 1 heaping teaspoon, and set them on the baking sheet about 1" apart. Bake until lightly browned, about 15 minutes.

4. Remove the baking sheet from the oven and place it on a rack, allowing the cookies to cool for 30 minutes. Transfer the cookies to a decorative plate and serve with fruit compote.

Makes 24 cookies, 2 per serving. Per serving: 74 calories, 1 g protein, 11 g carbohydrate, 2 g fat, trace fiber

Note: The macaroons will keep in a sealed container for several days.

Daisy's Chocolate-Covered Almonds

When a longtime patient of mine, Daisy Wing, heard that I like chocolate and nuts, she made me a batch of these delicious chocolate almond clusters. I enjoyed them so much that I talked her into divulging her technique. They make a wonderful low-glycemic-load dessert.

>   **1 pound raw almonds**
>   **½ pound semisweet chocolate**

1. Preheat the oven to 275°F. Spread the almonds evenly on a baking sheet.
2. Roast the almonds for 1 hour and 40 minutes. Stir them every 15 minutes, so they roast evenly. Remove them from the oven and let them cool.
3. Put the chocolate in a glass bowl and microwave on medium for 2 minutes, until melted.
4. While the almonds are still warm, mix them into the melted chocolate. Use a spoon to scoop out clusters of approximately 10 chocolate-covered almonds each. Use a spatula to scrape the clusters off the spoon onto a tray lined with waxed paper.
5. Allow the candy to cool until the chocolate is hard.

Makes approximately 4 dozen clusters. Per cluster: 164 calories, 2 g protein, 3 g carbohydrate, 5 g fat, 1 g fiber

Note: Store in an airtight container in the freezer for up to 6 months.

Raspberry-Studded Mini Cheesecakes with Pignoli Crust

Top off a low-glycemic-load meal with one of these and you're sure to feel well fed and satisfied. Instead of the standard graham cracker crust made with flour, these cheesecakes have a base of rich, fragrant pine nuts, called *pignoli* in Italian. While making mini cheesecakes takes more effort than baking just one big cake, it guarantees portion control—that is, if you don't eat a half dozen at once!

½ cup pine nuts
2 eggs, separated
12 ounces cream cheese, softened
5 tablespoons sugar, divided
Juice and peel of ½ lemon
1½ teaspoons all-purpose flour
1½ cups sour cream
1 teaspoon vanilla extract
24 fresh or frozen raspberries

1. Place 24 paper cup liners (1½" diameter) in the cups of a 24-cup muffin pan. Preheat the oven to 325°F.

2. Put the pine nuts in a food processor fitted with a metal blade and process for 3 to 4 seconds, until the nuts have the coarse texture of bread crumbs. Sprinkle the nuts into the muffin cups and manually press down to form a bottom crust for the cheesecakes.

3. In a medium bowl, using an electric mixer, beat the egg yolks until light. Add the cream cheese, 4 tablespoons of the sugar, and the lemon peel and juice. Beat until smooth. Stir in the flour.

4. Beat the egg whites until they hold soft peaks. Using a rubber spatula, fold the whites into the cheese mixture. Spoon the batter into the muffin tin. Place the tin in a water bath (see note on page 328). Carefully transfer to the oven. Bake until the cakes are very lightly browned and just set, about 50 minutes. Remove the cheesecakes and turn up the oven to 450°F.

(continued)

5. In a small bowl, combine the sour cream, the vanilla extract, and the remaining 1 tablespoon sugar. Spread over the top of each cheesecake. Return the muffin pan filled with cheesecakes to the oven, without the baking pan, and bake for 5 minutes. Remove the pan and set it on a rack to cool. Cover loosely with plastic wrap and refrigerate until well chilled.

6. To serve, insert a fresh raspberry into the center of each cheesecake. Alternatively, if using frozen berries, insert the berries in the warm cheesecakes before they cool, to defrost the fruit, and then refrigerate. (If the cheesecakes are to be eaten over several days, add the fruit just before serving.)

Makes 24 servings of 1 cheesecake. Per serving: 60 calories, 2 g protein, 3 g carbohydrate, 5 g fat, trace fiber

Note: A water bath promotes more even cooking. Use a baking pan larger than the muffin tin and place the tin in the pan. Add warm water to the baking pan until it comes at least halfway up the height of the muffin tin.

Warm Caramelized Pears with Roasted Pecans and Ice Cream

These pears are cooked in a butterscotch sauce that, as it cooks down, eventually caramelizes the pears. Add richly fragrant pecans, top the warm pears with a small amount of cool ice cream, and you have an intensely pleasurable dessert. This dish is easy to make. The only challenge is keeping to a modest portion. Remember, ¾ cup of ice cream is meant to serve six.

> **2 Bosc pears**
> **1 cup water**
> **2 tablespoons butterscotch topping**
> **Grated peel of ½ lemon (1 tablespoon)**
> **1 teaspoon butter**
> **¼ cup pecans**
> **¾ cup premium vanilla ice cream**

1. Halve the pears lengthwise and remove their cores. Cut each half lengthwise into narrow slices. Put the water and butterscotch in a medium saucepan and stir to combine. Add the pears and lemon peel.

2. Cook the pears over medium heat, stirring occasionally. After about 30 minutes, the pears will have reduced in size, and most of the cooking liquid will have evaporated. Continue cooking until the remaining sauce is very thick and begins to coat the fruit, an additional 10 minutes.

3. Meanwhile, put the butter in a small skillet; add the pecans and toast over medium heat, stirring frequently, until they become fragrant, about 5 minutes. Remove from the heat and set aside.

4. To assemble the dessert, place 3 or 4 pear slices on a salad plate or in a stemmed glass. Using a spoon slightly larger than a standard flatware teaspoon, scoop a spoonful of ice cream on top of the warm pear and sprinkle with a few pecans. Proceed with the other servings, or refrigerate the remaining pears and pecans for later use.

6 servings. Per serving: 130 calories, 2 g protein, 18 g carbohydrate, 7 g fat, 2 g fiber

Appendix A

Glycemic Loads of Common Foods

Food Item	Description	Available Carbohydrate (percent)	Typical American Serving	Glycemic Load
Baked Goods				
Oatmeal cookie	1 medium	68	1 oz	102
Apple muffin, sugarless	2½" diameter	32	2½ oz	107
Cookie, average, all types	1 medium	64	1 oz	114
Croissant	1 medium	46	1½ oz	127
Crumpet	1 medium	38	2 oz	148
Bran muffin	2½" diameter	42	2 oz	149
Pastry	Average serving	46	2 oz	149
Chocolate cake	1 slice (4" × 4" × 1")	47	3 oz	154
Vanilla wafers	4 wafers	72	1 oz	159
Graham cracker	1 rectangle	72	1 oz	159
Blueberry muffin	2½" diameter	51	2 oz	169
Pita bread	1 medium	57	2 oz	189
Carrot cake	1 square (3" × 3" × 1½")	56	2 oz	199
Carrot muffin	2½" diameter	56	2 oz	199
Waffle	7" diameter	37	2½ oz	203
Doughnut	1 medium	49	2 oz	205

Food Item	Description	Available Carbohydrate (percent)	Typical American Serving	Glycemic Load
Baked Goods (continued)				
Cupcake	2½" diameter	68	1½ oz	213
Angel food cake	1 slice (4" × 4" × 1")	58	2 oz	216
English muffin	1 medium	47	2 oz	224
Pound cake	1 slice (4" × 4" × 1")	53	3 oz	241
Corn muffin	2½" diameter	51	2 oz	299
Pancake	5" diameter	73	2½ oz	346
Alcoholic Beverages				
Spirits	1½ oz	0	1½ oz	<15
Red wine	6 oz glass	0	6 oz	<15
White wine	6 oz glass	0	6 oz	<15
Beer	12 oz can/bottle	3	12 oz	70
Nonalcoholic Beverages				
Tomato juice	6 oz glass	4	6 oz	27
V8 juice	6 oz glass	4	6 oz	27
Carrot juice	6 oz glass	12	6 oz	68
Grapefruit juice, unsweetened	6 oz glass	9	6 oz	75
Apple juice, unsweetened	6 oz glass	12	6 oz	82
Chocolate milk	8 oz glass	10	8 oz	82
Orange juice	6 oz glass	10	6 oz	89
Prune juice	6 oz glass	14	6 oz	102
Cranberry juice	6 oz glass	12	6 oz	109
Pineapple juice, unsweetened	6 oz glass	14	6 oz	109
Raspberry smoothie	8 oz glass	16	8 oz	127
Lemonade	8 oz glass	11	8 oz	136
Ensure	8 oz glass	17	8 oz	182

Food Item	Description	Available Carbohydrate (percent)	Typical American Serving	Glycemic Load
Nonalcoholic Beverages (continued)				
Coca-Cola	12 oz can	10	12 oz	218
Gatorade	20 oz bottle	6	20 oz	273
Orange soda	12 oz glass	14	12 oz	314
Breads and Rolls				
Tortilla (wheat)	1 medium	52	1⅜ oz	64
Pizza crust	1 slice	22	3½ oz	70
Tortilla (corn)	1 medium	48	1¼ oz	87
White bread	½" slice	47	1 oz	107
Whole meal rye bread	⅜" slice	40	2 oz	114
Sourdough bread	⅜" slice	47	1½ oz	114
Oat bran bread	⅜" slice	60	1½ oz	128
Whole wheat bread	½" slice	43	1½ oz	129
Rye bread	⅜" slice	47	1½ oz	142
Banana bread, sugarless	1 slice (4" × 4" × 1")	48	3 oz	170
80% whole kernel oat bread	⅜" slice	63	1½ oz	170
Buckwheat bread	⅜" slice	63	1½ oz	183
80% whole kernel barley bread	⅜" slice	67	1½ oz	185
Pita bread	8" diameter	57	2 oz	189
Hamburger bun	Top & bottom, 5" diameter	50	2½ oz	213
80% whole kernel wheat bread	⅜" slice	67	2¼ oz	213
French bread	½" slice	50	2 oz	284
Bagel	1 medium	50	3⅓ oz	340
Breakfast Cereals				
All-Bran	½ c	77	1 oz	85
Muesli	1 c	53	1 oz	95

Food Item	Description	Available Carbohydrate (percent)	Typical American Serving	Glycemic Load
Breakfast Cereals (continued)				
Oatmeal (from rolled oats)	1 c	10	8 oz	123
Special K	1 c	70	1 oz	133
Cheerios	1 c	40	1 oz	142
Shredded wheat	1 c	67	1 oz	142
Grape-Nuts	1 c	70	1 oz	142
Granola	1 c	87	1 oz	142
Puffed wheat	1 c	70	1 oz	151
Kashi	1 c	80	1 oz	151
Instant oatmeal	1 c	10	8 oz	154
Cream of Wheat, cooked	1 c	10	8 oz	154
Total	1 c	73	1 oz	161
Froot Loops	1 c	87	1 oz	170
Cornflakes	1 c	77	1 oz	199
Rice Krispies	1 c	87	1 oz	208
Rice Chex	1 c	87	1 oz	218
Raisin bran	1 c	63	2 oz	227
Candy and Snacks				
Sugar-free milk chocolate	2 squares (1" × 1" × ¼")	30	1 oz	17
Life Saver	1 piece	100	¹⁄₁₀ oz	20
Dark chocolate	2 squares (1" × 1" × ¼")	52	1 oz	44
Peanut M&Ms	1 snack-size package	57	¾ oz	43
Licorice	1 twist	70	⅓ oz	45
White chocolate	2 squares (1" × 1" × ¼")	44	⅔ oz	49
Milk chocolate	2 squares (1" × 1" × ¼")	44	1 oz	68
Jelly beans	6 beans	93	½ oz	104

Food Item	Description	Available Carbohydrate (percent)	Typical American Serving	Glycemic Load
Candy and Snacks (continued)				
Granola bar, apple or cranberry	1 bar	77	1 oz	131
Snickers bar	1 regular-size bar	57	2 oz	218
Chips and Crackers				
Potato chips	Small bag	42	1 oz	62
Corn chips	1 package	52	1 oz	97
Popcorn	4 cups	55	1 oz	114
Rye crisp	1 rectangle	64	1 oz	125
Wheat Thins	4 small	68	1 oz	136
Soda crackers	2 regular size	68	1 oz	136
Pretzels	Small bag	67	1 oz	151
Rice cakes	3 regular size	84	1 oz	190
Dairy Products				
Cheese	2" × 2" × 1" slice	0	2 oz	<15
Butter	1 Tbsp	0	¼ oz	<15
Margarine	Typical serving	0	¼ oz	<15
Sour cream	Typical serving	0	2 oz	<15
Yogurt, full fat (unsweetened)	½ c	5	4 oz	17
Milk (whole)	8 oz glass	5	8 oz	37
Milk (fat free)	8 oz glass	5	8 oz	41
Yogurt, low fat (sweetened)	½ c	16	4 oz	57
Soy milk	8 oz glass	7	8 oz	62
Vanilla ice cream (high fat)	½ c	18	4 oz	68
Milk (low-fat chocolate)	8 oz glass	10	8 oz	82
Custard	½ c	17	4½ oz	89
Chocolate pudding	½ c	16	4½ oz	89
Chocolate ice cream (high fat)	½ c	18	4½ oz	91

Food Item	Description	Available Carbohydrate (percent)	Typical American Serving	Glycemic Load
Dairy Products (continued)				
Vanilla ice cream (low fat)	½ c	36	4 oz	159
Frozen tofu	½ c	30	4 oz	379
Fruit				
Strawberries	1 c	3	5½ oz	13
Apricot	1 medium	8	2 oz	24
Grapefruit	1 half	9	4½ oz	32
Plum	1 medium	10	3 oz	36
Nectarine	1 medium	8	4 oz	38
Cherries, dark	8	12	2 oz	43
Kiwifruit	1 medium	10	3 oz	43
Peaches, canned in natural juice	½ c	10	4 oz	45
Peach, fresh	1 medium	9	4 oz	47
Grapes	½ c	15	2½ oz	47
Pineapple	1 slice (¾" × 3½" wide)	11	3 oz	50
Watermelon	1 c cubed	5	5½ oz	52
Cantaloupe	1 c cubed	5	5½ oz	52
Pear	1 medium	9	6 oz	57
Mango	½ c	14	3 oz	57
Orange	1 medium	9	6 oz	71
Apricot, dried	2 oz	45	2 oz	76
Apple	1 medium	13	5½ oz	78
Banana	1 medium	17	3¼ oz	85
Prunes, pitted, dried	2 oz	55	2 oz	95
Apple, dried	2 oz	60	2 oz	104
Peaches, canned in heavy syrup	½ c	16	4 oz	112
Raisins	2 Tbsp	73	1 oz	133
Figs	3 medium	43	2 oz	151
Dates	5 medium	67	1½ oz	298

Food Item	Description	Available Carbohydrate (percent)	Typical American Serving	Glycemic Load
Meat				
Beef	10 oz steak	0	10 oz	<15
Pork	Two 5 oz chops	0	10 oz	<15
Chicken	1 breast	0	10 oz	<15
Fish	8 oz fillet	0	8 oz	<15
Lamb	Three 4 oz chops	0	12 oz	<15
Mixed Meals				
Deluxe burger, no bun	1 medium	16	3¼ oz	<15
Pizza, minus outer rim of crust	1 slice	12	3 oz	45
Wheat tortilla, bean filled	1 burrito	18	4 oz	50
Chicken nuggets	4 oz	16	4 oz	70
Deluxe burger minus top bun	1 medium	8	4¼ oz	80
Cannelloni, spinach, ricotta	2 tubes	18	12 oz	88
Pizza, crust intact	1 slice	24	4 oz	90
Chili con carne	1 cup	12	8 oz	91
Veggie burger	1 medium	24	3½ oz	140
Deluxe hamburger	1 medium	16	5¾ oz	170
Fillet-O-Fish sandwich	1 medium	30	4½ oz	200
Chicken korma and rice	10 oz	16	10 oz	210
McChicken sandwich	1 medium	22	6½ oz	260
Nuts				
Peanuts	¼ c	8	1¼ oz	<15
Walnuts	¼ c	8	1¼ oz	<15
Almonds	¼ c	8	1¼ oz	<15
Cashews	¼ c	26	1¼ oz	21

Food Item	Description	Available Carbohydrate (percent)	Typical American Serving	Glycemic Load
Pasta				
Asian bean noodles	1 c	25	5 oz	118
Spaghetti, whole grain	1 c	23	5 oz	126
Vermicelli	1 c	24	5 oz	126
Spaghetti (boiled 5 min)	1 c	27	5 oz	142
Fettuccine	1 c	23	5 oz	142
Noodles (instant, boiled 2 min)	1 c	22	5 oz	150
Capellini	1 c	25	5 oz	158
Spaghetti (boiled 10–15 min)	1 c	27	5 oz	166
Linguine	1 c	25	5 oz	181
Macaroni	1 c	28	5 oz	181
Rice noodles	1 c	22	5 oz	181
Spaghetti (boiled 20 min)	1 c	24	5 oz	213
Macaroni and cheese (boxed)	1 c	28	5 oz	252
Gnocchi	1 c	27	5 oz	260
Soups				
Tomato soup	1 c	7	8 oz	55
Minestrone	1 c	7	8 oz	64
Lentil soup	1 c	8	8 oz	82
Split pea soup	1 c	11	8 oz	145
Black bean soup	1 c	11	8 oz	154
Sweeteners				
Artificial sweeteners	1 tsp		⅙ oz	<15
Honey	1 tsp	72	⅙ oz	16
Table sugar	1 rounded tsp	100	⅙ oz	28
Syrup	¼ c	100	2 oz	364

Food Item	Description	Available Carbohydrate (percent)	Typical American Serving	Glycemic Load
Vegetables				
Lettuce	1 c	3	2½ oz	<15
Spinach	1 c	5	2½ oz	<15
Cucumber	1 c	2	6 oz	<15
Mushrooms	½ c	7	2 oz	<15
Asparagus	4 spears	6	3 oz	<15
Peppers	½ medium	4	2 oz	<15
Broccoli	½ c	6	1½ oz	<15
Carrot (raw)	1 medium (7½")	10	3 oz	11
Tomato	1 medium	6	5 oz	<15
Chickpeas, boiled	2 Tbsp	10	1 oz	<15
Peas	¼ c	9	1½ oz	16
Chickpeas, boiled	½ c	20	3 oz	17
Carrots, boiled	⅔ c	6	3 oz	21
Fava beans	½ c	6	3 oz	32
Lentils	½ c	11	3½ oz	33
Butter beans	½ c	13	3 oz	34
Cannellini beans	½ c	14	3 oz	34
Kidney beans	½ c	17	3 oz	40
Navy beans	½ c	10	3 oz	40
Parsnips	½ c	10	3 oz	50
Lima beans	½ c	12	3 oz	57
Refried pinto beans	½ c	17	3 oz	57
Black-eyed peas	½ c	20	3 oz	74
Yam	½ c	24	5 oz	123
Quinoa	1 c	17	6½ oz	160
Potato, instant mashed	¾ c	13	5 oz	161
Sweet potato	½ c	19	5 oz	161
Corn on the cob	1 ear	21	5⅓ oz	171
Couscous	½ c	23	4 oz	174
Rice cakes	1 medium	84	1 oz	193
French fries	Medium serving (McDonald's)	19	5¼ oz	219

Food Item	Description	Available Carbohydrate (percent)	Typical American Serving	Glycemic Load
Vegetables (continued)				
Brown and wild rice mix	1 c	26	6½ oz	221
Brown rice	1 c	22	6½ oz	222
Baked potato	1 medium	20	5 oz	246
Basmati rice	1 c	25	6½ oz	271
White rice	1 c	24	6½ oz	283
Sticky white rice	1 c	19	6½ oz	295
Miscellaneous				
Eggs	Typical serving	0	1½ oz	<15
Salad dressing	Typical serving	10	2 oz	<15
Agave	2 tsp	100	¼ oz	<15
Cane sugar	1 level tsp	100	⅛ oz	28

Appendix B

2-Week Low-Glycemic-Load Meal Plan

R emember: Your goal is to keep the daily sum of your glycemic loads (GL) below 500.

Note: Glycemic loads estimated to be less than 20 are not listed.

Monday

Breakfast (Dr. Thompson's Personal 4-Minute, 30-Second Power Breakfast)

Eggs Puttanesca (page 162)
½ High-Fiber Bran Muffin (GL 60) (page 173)
Starbucks Via instant coffee

Lunch

Strawberries dipped in 1 tsp sugar (GL 30)
Salad Niçoise (page 195)
1 slice of French bread (GL 100)
Butter
Coffee or tea

Dinner

Middle Eastern/Southwestern Fusion Salad (page 207)
Southwestern Pork with Peach Salsa (page 289)

Fauxtatoes (GL 50) (page 223)
Broccoli (GL 15)
Milk or red wine (GL 30)
Dessert: 10 Ghirardelli 60% Cacao Bittersweet Chocolate
    Chips (GL 60)
Estimated Glycemic Load for the Day: 345

Tuesday

Breakfast

Breakfast Cereal Sundae (GL 60) (page 166)
Coffee or tea

Lunch

½ apple, sliced (GL 35)
Turkey and avocado flour tortilla wrap (GL 85)
Milk or diet soda (GL 30)

Dinner

Iceberg wedge salad
Easy and Elegant Salmon Packets (page 301)
Orange-Hazelnut Green Beans (GL 20) (page 236)
Buttered potato skins (GL 60)
Milk or white wine (GL 30)
Dessert: 3 clusters Daisy's Chocolate-Covered Almonds
    (GL 45) (page 326)
Estimated Glycemic Load for the Day: 365

Wednesday

Breakfast

Sliced peach and cream (GL 50)
Homemade Breakfast Burrito (GL 70) (page 150)
Coffee or tea

Lunch

Grilled Chicken Salad with Spinach and Apples (page 215)
8 potato chips (GL 70)
Coffee, tea, or milk (GL 30)

Dinner (out at a pizza parlor)

Romaine, sliced olive, and grated Parmesan cheese salad with
    blue cheese dressing
3 slices sausage-mushroom pizza (outer third of crust
    removed) (GL 60)
Diet soda or red wine
Dessert: Dark chocolate, two 1" squares (GL 60)

Estimated Glycemic Load for the Day: 340

Thursday

Breakfast

⅓ c bran cereal with chopped walnuts, strawberries, and milk
    (GL 85)
Coffee, tea, or milk (GL 30)

Lunch

Side salad
Curried Coconut Cream of Chicken Soup (GL 60) (page 250)
Coffee, tea, or milk (GL 30)

Dinner

Fruit Salad with Poppy Seed Dressing (GL 70) (page 209)
Ginger-Sesame Glazed Chicken (page 260)
Broccoli with butter and lemon juice (GL 20)
Rice-a-Phony (GL 30) (page 226)
White wine or milk (GL 30)
Dessert: Daisy's Chocolate-Covered Almonds (GL 60)
    (page 326)

Estimated Glycemic Load for the Day: 415

Friday

Breakfast
Yogurt Parfait (GL 60) (page 168)
½ High-Fiber Bran Muffin (GL 60) (page 173)
Coffee or tea

Lunch
French onion soup
Chicken–Smoked Gouda Salad (page 212)
Coffee, tea, or milk (GL 30)

Dinner
Vietnamese Cucumber Salad (page 208)
Grilled swordfish
Asparagus
½ c wild rice (GL 90)
Dessert: ¼ c gourmet ice cream (GL 40)
Estimated Glycemic Load for the Day: 280

Saturday

Breakfast
½ c yogurt (GL 20)
Blueberries
Spinach-Mushroom Frittata (GL 30) (page 152)
Coffee or tea

Lunch
Peach (GL 50)
Turkey, ham, and Swiss cheese wrap (GL 85)
Coffee, tea, or diet soda

Dinner (barbecue)
Caesar salad
Rib-eye steak
Chipotle Mushrooms (page 232)
½ baked potato with butter and sour cream (GL 130)
Red wine or milk (GL 30)

Dessert: Dark chocolate (two 1" squares) (GL 60)

Estimated Glycemic Load for the Day: 405

Sunday

Breakfast

½ grapefruit (GL 30)
Avocado, Bacon, and Spinach Omelet (page 158)
Coffee or tea

Lunch

4 soda crackers (GL 60)
Seriously Simple Southwestern Sausage Soup (page 255)
Coffee, tea, or milk (GL 30)

Dinner

Lettuce, avocado, tomato, and red bell pepper salad with
    vinaigrette
Shrimp with Garlic, Chile, and Herbs (page 304)
Black beans cooked with a clove of garlic (GL 50)
White wine or milk (GL 30)
Dessert: 8 cinnamon jelly beans (GL 60)

Estimated Glycemic Load for the Day: 260

Monday

Breakfast

½ grapefruit (GL 30)
Eggs Puttanesca (page 162)
½ High-Fiber Bran Muffin (GL 60) (page 173)
Coffee, tea, or milk (GL 30)

Lunch

½ apple, sliced (GL 35)
Curried Coconut Cream of Chicken Soup (page 250)
Coffee, tea, or milk (GL 30)

Dinner

Simple dinner salad (lettuce, tomato, leeks, blue cheese
   dressing)
Pork chops with Molly's Piquant Onion Relish (page 197)
Fauxtatoes (GL 30) (page 223)
Stir-Fried Snow Peas with Water Chestnuts and Cashews
   (GL 30) (page 231)
Red wine or milk (GL 30)
Dessert: ¼ c gourmet ice cream (GL 40)

Estimated Glycemic Load for the Day: 315

Tuesday

Breakfast

½ c strawberries and ¼ c yogurt (GL 20)
Cinnamon, Flax, and Bran Granola (GL 60) (page 175)
Coffee or tea

Lunch

Chopped salad (romaine, turkey, avocado, blue cheese
   crumbles)
Dark chocolate (two 1" squares) (GL 50)
Coffee, tea, or milk (GL 30)

Dinner

Easy Pea Salad (GL 30) (page 206)
Weeknight Fish Stew (page 312)
4 Sunflower-Cornmeal Cheese Crackers (GL 40) (page 182)
White wine or milk (GL 30)
Dessert: 3 clusters Daisy's Chocolate-Covered Almonds
   (GL 45) (page 326)

Estimated Glycemic Load for the Day: 305

Wednesday

Breakfast

½ orange, sliced (GL 35)
Savory Scramble (page 161)
Coffee or tea

Lunch

1 slice of bread (GL 100)
Butter
Walnut-Chicken Salad (page 218)
Dark chocolate (two 1" squares) (GL 50)
Coffee, tea, or milk (GL 30)

Dinner

Greek salad (cucumber, tomato, feta cheese, olive oil,
    vinegar)
Broiled or barbecued lamb chops
Cauliflower-Potato Mash (GL 60) (page 224)
Red wine or milk (GL 30)
Dessert: Warm Caramelized Pears with Roasted Pecans and
    Ice Cream (GL 60) (page 329)
Estimated Glycemic Load for the Day: 365

Thursday

Breakfast

½ apple, sliced (GL 40)
Apple, Cheddar, and Bacon Omelet (page 157)
Coffee or tea

Lunch

Simple lettuce and tomato side salad with blue cheese or
    ranch dressing
Easy Chicken Gumbo (page 251)
Coffee, tea, or milk (GL 30)

Dinner (out at a diner)

Wedge salad, ranch dressing, blue cheese crumbles
Large pickle
Cheeseburger (top of bun removed) (GL 70)
8 potato chips (GL 70)
Dark chocolate (two 1" squares) (GL 50)
Diet soda or beer (GL 70)

Estimated Glycemic Load for the Day: 330

Friday

Breakfast

½ grapefruit (GL 30)
Scrambled eggs and sausage
½ High-Fiber Bran Muffin (GL 60) (page 173)
Coffee or tea

Lunch

Chicken–Smoked Gouda Salad (page 212)
Red Bell Pepper Soup Topped with Sour Cream (page 257)
Coffee, tea, or milk (GL 30)

Dinner

Baked salmon
Broccoli with Cashews (page 230)
Rice-a-Phony (GL 30) (page 226)
White wine or milk (GL 30)
Dessert: ¼ c gourmet ice cream and strawberries (GL 50)

Estimated Glycemic Load for the Day: 230

Saturday

Breakfast

Sliced kiwifruit (GL 40)
Zucchini-Pepper Frittata (page 154)
1 slice buttered toast sprinkled with cinnamon and Splenda
    (GL 100)
Coffee or tea

Lunch

Lettuce, tomato, and avocado salad
Easy Chicken Gumbo (page 251)
Coffee, tea, or milk (GL 30)

Dinner

Sliced tomato, cucumber, and vinegar salad
Savory Greek Lamb Shanks and Lima Beans (GL 30)
    (page 294)
½ baked sweet potato (GL 80)
Red wine or milk (GL 30)
Dessert: Raspberry-Studded Mini Cheesecake with Pignoli
    Crust (page 327)
Estimated Glycemic Load for the Day: 310

Sunday

Breakfast

Berries and yogurt (GL 30)
Apple-Walnut Pancake (GL 20) (page 180)
Coffee, tea, or milk (GL 30)

Lunch

Apple (GL 70)
Almonds
Assorted cheeses
Coffee, tea, or diet soda

Dinner

Coleslaw (page 203)
Classic Unpotato Salad (GL 30) (page 205)
Fried chicken
Coffee, tea, or milk (GL 30)
Dessert: 8 cinnamon jelly beans (GL 60)
Estimated Glycemic Load for the Day: 270

Appendix C

References

Aude, Y. W., et al. 2004. The national cholesterol education program diet v. a diet lower in carbohydrates and higher in protein and monounsaturated fat: A randomized trial. *Archives of Internal Medicine* 164: 2141–46.

Baer, D. J., et al. 1997. Dietary fiber decreases the metabolizable energy content and nutrient digestibility of mixed diets fed to humans. *Journal of Nutrition* 127 (4): 579–86.

Bond-Brill, J., et al. 2002. Dose-response effect of walking exercise on weight loss: How much is enough? *International Journal of Obesity and Related Metabolic Disorders* 26 (11): 1484–93.

Brand-Miller, J. D., et al. 2003. Physiological validation of the concept of glycemic load in lean young adults. *Journal of Nutrition* 133 (9): 2728–32.

Bryner, R. W., et al. 1999. Effects of resistance versus aerobic training combined with an 800 calorie liquid diet on lean body mass and resting metabolic rate. *Journal of the American College of Nutrition* 18 (2): 115–21.

Di Meglio, D. P., and R. D. Mattes. 2000. Liquid versus solid carbohydrate: Effects on food intake and body weight. *International Journal of Obesity and Related Metabolic Disorders* 24 (6): 794–800.

Flegal, K. M., et al. 2002. Prevalence and trends in obesity among US adults, 1999–2000. *Journal of the American Medical Association* 288: 1728–32.

Fontaine, K. R., et al. 2003. Years of life lost due to obesity. *Journal of the American Medical Association* 289 (2): 187–93.

Foster, G. D., et al. 2003. A randomized trial of a low-carbohydrate diet for obesity. *New England Journal of Medicine* 348 (21): 2082–90.

Foster-Powell, K., S. H. A. Holt, and J. D. Brand-Miller. 2002. International table of glycemic index and glycemic load values. *American Journal of Clinical Nutrition* 76: 5–6.

Hays, J. H., et al. 2003. Effects of a high saturated fat and no-starch diet on serum lipid subfractions in patients with documented atherosclerotic cardiovascular disease. *Mayo Clinic Proceedings* 78: 1331–36.

Howard, B. V., et al. 2006. Low fat dietary pattern and risk of cardiovascular disease. *Journal of the American Medical Association* 295 (6): 655–66.

Irwin, M. L., et al. 2003. Effect of exercise on total and intra-abdominal body fat in postmenopausal women: A randomized controlled trial. *Journal of the American Medical Association* 289 (3): 323–30.

Jarvi, A. E., et al. 1999. Improved glycemic control and lipid profile and normalized fibrinolytic activity on a low-glycemic index diet in type 2 diabetic patients. *Diabetes Care* 22 (1): 10–18.

Lavin, J. H., et al. 2002. An investigation of the role of oro-sensory stimulation in sugar satiety. *International Journal of Obesity and Related Metabolic Disorders* 26 (3): 384–88.

Manson, J. E., et al. 2002. Walking compared with vigorous exercise for the prevention of cardiovascular events in women. *New England Journal of Medicine* 347 (10): 716–25.

Mattes, R. D., and D. Rothacker. 2001. Beverage viscosity is inversely related to postprandial hunger in humans. *Physiological Behavior* 74 (4–5): 551–57.

Miyatake, N., et al. 2002. Daily walking reduces visceral adipose tissue areas and improves insulin resistance in Japanese obese subjects. *Diabetes Research in Clinical Practice* 58 (2): 101–7.

National Center for Health Statistics. 2001. Third National Health and Nutrition Examination Survey. www.cdc.gov/nchs/nhanes.htm (search "body weight").

O'Keefe, J. H., and L. Cordain. 2004. Cardiovascular disease resulting from a diet and lifestyle at odds with our Paleolithic genome: How to become a 21st-century hunter-gatherer. *Mayo Clinic Proceedings* 79: 101–8.

Packianathan, I. C., et al. 2002. The eating disorder inventory in a UK National Health Service obesity clinic and its response to modest weight loss. *Eating Behavior* 3 (3): 275–84.

Pasman, W. J., et al. 2003. Effect of two breakfasts, different in carbohydrate composition, on hunger and satiety and mood in healthy men. *International Journal of Obesity and Related Metabolic Disorders* 27 (6): 663–68.

Pelkman, C. L., et al. 2004. Effects of moderate-fat (from mono-unsaturated fat) and low-fat weight-loss diets on the serum lipid profile in overweight and obese men and women. *American Journal of Clinical Nutrition* 79: 204–12.

Pereira, M. A. 2002. Dairy consumption, obesity, and the insulin resistance syndrome in young adults: The CARDIA study. *Journal of the American Medical Association* 287 (16): 2081–89.

Pereira, M. A., et al. 2004. Effects of a low-glycemic load diet on resting energy expenditure and heart disease risk factors during weight loss. *Journal of the American Medical Association* 292 (20): 2482–90.

Petersen, K. F., et al. 2004. Impaired mitochondrial activity in the insulin-resistant offspring of patients with type 2 diabetes. *New England Journal of Medicine* 350: 664–71.

Ryden, A., et al. 2003. Severe obesity and personality: A comparative controlled study of personality traits. *International Journal of Obesity and Related Metabolic Disorders* 27 (12): 1534–40.

Samaha, F. F., et al. 2003. A low-carbohydrate as compared with a low-fat diet for severe obesity. *New England Journal of Medicine* 348 (21): 2082–90.

Schulze, M. B. 2004. Sugar-sweetened beverages, weight gain, and incidence of type 2 diabetes in young and middle-aged women. *Journal of the American Medical Association* 292 (8): 927–35.

Slentz, C. A., et al. 2004. Effects of the amount of exercise on body weight, body composition, and measures of central obesity. *Archives of Internal Medicine* 164: 31–39.

Sparti, A., et al. 2000. Effects of a diet high or low in unavailable and slowly digested carbohydrates on the pattern of 24 hour substrate oxidation and feelings of hunger in humans. *American Journal of Clinical Nutrition* 72 (6): 1461–68.

Sturm, R. 2003. Increases in clinically severe obesity in the United States 1986–2000. *Archives of Internal Medicine* 163: 2146–48.

Taylor, R. 2004. Causation of type 2 diabetes: The Gordian knot unravels. *New England Journal of Medicine* 350: 639–41.

Tuomilehto, J., et al. 2004. Coffee consumption and risk of type 2 diabetes mellitus among middle-aged Finnish men and women. *Journal of the American Medical Association* 291 (10): 1213–19.

United States Department of Agriculture, Agricultural Research Service. 2004. National Nutrient Database for Standard Reference, Release 17. Nutrient Data Laboratory Home Page, www.nal.usda.gov/fnic/foodcomp.

Van Wymelbeke, V., et al. 2004. Influence of repeated consumption of beverages containing sucrose or intense sweeteners on food intake. *European Journal of Clinical Nutrition* 58 (1): 154–61.

Warren, J. M., et al. 2003. Low glycemic index breakfasts and reduced food intake in preadolescent children. *Pediatrics* 112 (5): e414.

Watkins, L. L., et al. 2003. Effects of exercise and weight loss on cardiac risk factors associated with Syndrome X. *Archives of Internal Medicine* 163: 1889–95.

Westerterp, K. R., and A. D. Kester. 2003. Physical activity in confined conditions as an indicator of free-living physical activity. *Obesity Research* 11 (7): 865–68.

Appendix D

Web Sites

- www.lowglycemicload.com This is a supplement to the book. You will find updated glucose-load tables, the latest research, additional information on such topics as medications, and more recipes. You can also submit questions and comments about your experience with low glycemic eating.
- http://www.heart.org/HEARTORG/Conditions/The-Heart-Profilers_UCM_304738_Article.jsp An interactive tool provided by the American Heart Association for helping people make informed decisions about high blood cholesterol, high blood pressure, and several heart conditions.
- www.holdthetoast.com An excellent source for low glycemic meals and snacks by Dana Carpender, author of *500 Low-Carb Recipes: 500 Recipes, from Snacks to Desserts, That the Whole Family Will Love.*
- www.atkins.com This Web site contains hundreds of recipes for low-carbohydrate dishes.
- www.sugarbusters.com Delicious low-glycemic-load dishes.

Index

Underscored references indicate tables or boxed text.

Restaurants *(cont.)*
    Japanese, 133
    Mexican, 133–34
    pizza parlors, 134
    seafood, 134–35
    standard American, 131
    steak houses, 135
    tips for eating at, 130–31
Rice
    as "comfort food," 125
    glucose shocks from, 38–39
    increased consumption of (1970 vs.
        1997), 25, 25
    reducing intake of, 16, 57
    substitutes for, 225–28
    wild, 228
Rice protein powder, 140
Rickets, 22
Ricotta cheese, 222
Romano cheese, 152–53, 215, 238
Rosemary, 292
Ruby Tuesday, 131

S**alads**
    for avoiding glucose shock, 59
    convenience foods, 129
    dressings
        Apricot-Mustard Dressing, 213
        Balsamic-Mustard Sauce, 204
        basic vinaigrette, 193
        bottled, cautions for, 193
        Honey-Mustard Dressing, 214
        Poppy Seed Dressing, 209
        Strawberry Vinaigrette, 202
    glycemic load negligible for, 192
    popular, low-glycemic-load, 192–94
    recipes
        Beet and Pear Salad with Warm
            Breaded Goat Cheese, 200–201
        Chicken Slaw with Honey-Mustard
            Dressing, 214
        Chicken–Smoked Gouda Salad,
            212
        Classic Unpotato Salad, 205
        Coleslaw, 203
        Colorful Dill Egg Salad, 211
        Easy Pea Salad, 206
        Fruit Salad with Poppy Seed Dressing,
            209
        Grilled Chicken Salad with Spinach
            and Apples, 215
        Ham and Pineapple Slaw, 220
        Middle Eastern/Southwestern Fusion
            Salad, 207
        Molly's Piquant Onion Relish, 197
        Oriental Chicken Salad, 216–17
        Salad Niçoise, 195–96
        Strawberry Salad, 202

Tomatoes Stuffed with Curried Tuna
    Salad, 210
Vietnamese Cucumber Salad, 208
Walnut-Chicken Salad, 218–19
Warm Sweet and Sour Pork Salad,
    198–99
Salmon, 165, 301, 311
Salsa
    Cranberry Salsa, 267
    Seriously Simple Southwestern Sausage
        Soup, 255
    Southwestern Pork with Peach Salsa, 289
    Tomato-Corn Salsa, 244
Salt, 116
Sandwiches, replacing with wraps, 59–60
Saturated fats, 99–100
Sauces. *See also* Salsa
    Balsamic-Mustard Sauce, 204
    Ginger-Lime Dipping Sauce, 298
    Horseradish Sauce, 275
    Red Bell Pepper–Sun-Dried Tomato
        Sauce, 300
    Sour Cream–Roasted Red Bell Pepper
        Sauce, 302
Sausage
    Frenchified Meat Loaf, 274
    Homemade Breakfast Burrito, 150–51
    Jersey Girl Chili, 273
    Seriously Simple Southwestern Sausage
        Soup, 255
Scallions, pork with, 288
Scallops, 305–6
Scrambled eggs, 160–61
Seafood. *See* Fish and seafood
Seafood restaurants, 134–35
Seeds and nuts
    benefits of nuts, 59
    chocolate-covered nuts, 314
    nuts for balancing fat in diet, 104
    recipes
        Almond Cookies from Mix, 317
        Apple-Walnut Pancakes, 180–81
        Blue Cheese Walnut Pesto Chicken
            with Noodles, 264
        Broccoli and Almonds, 222
        Broccoli with Cashews, 230
        Cashew-Crusted Chicken, 262
        Chicken Slaw with Honey-Mustard
            Dressing, 214
        Cinnamon, Flax, and Bran Granola,
            175–76
        Daisy's Chocolate-Covered Almonds,
            326
        Flax Pancakes, 178
        Fruit Salad with Poppy Seed Dressing,
            209
        Green Beans with Pine Nuts, 235
        High-Fiber Bran Muffins, 173–74

taste satisfied by, 78
tips for making friends with, 78–80
Summer squash
   Cumin Grilled Zucchini with Tomato-
      Corn Salsa, 244–45
   Scalloped Summer Squash, 222
   Zucchini-Pepper Frittata, 154
Sunflower seeds, 175–76, 182, 184
Super Xers, 12–13
Sweets, choosing, 78–80. *See also* Sugar
Swiss cheese, 165, 310
Syndrome X, 8, 12–13. *See also* Insulin
   resistance

Taco Bell, 133
Tea, 71–72
T.G.I. Friday's, 131
Thrifty-gene hypothesis, 10
Thyroxin, 5
Tomatoes
   Baked Perch in Roasted Red Bell
      Pepper–Sun-Dried Tomato Sauce,
      300
   Cheese-Stuffed Peppers Two Ways, 243
   Cumin Grilled Zucchini with Tomato-
      Corn Salsa, 244–45
   Easy Chicken Gumbo, 251
   Homemade Breakfast Burrito, 150–51
   Jersey Girl Chili, 273
   Middle Eastern/Southwestern Fusion
      Salad, 207
   Red Bell Pepper Soup Topped with Sour
      Cream, 257
   Ricotta Tomatoes, 222
   Shrimp with Garlic, Chile, and Herbs,
      304
   Smoked Turkey, Sun-Dried Tomato, and
      Yellow Bell Pepper Pizza, 266
   Super-Chunky Slow-Cooker Vegetable-
      Beef Soup, 256
   Tomato and Mozzarella Salad, 193
   Tomatoes Stuffed with Curried Tuna
      Salad, 210
   Weeknight Fish Stew, 312
Tortillas
   low-carb, about, 143
   low-carb, commercial, 170
   recipes
      Homemade Breakfast Burrito, 150–51
      Hot Tuna Wraps, 310
      Smoked Turkey, Sun-Dried Tomato,
         and Yellow Bell Pepper Pizza, 266
   sandwich bread compared to, 60
Toxins
   in the news, 18
   starch, 19–20, 22–23
Trans fats, 102–3
Triceps press, 90

Triglyceride levels
   as insulin resistance indicator, 12
   lowered by Atkins diet, 34
   lowered by relieving insulin resistance,
      123
   in Super Xers, 13
Tuna
   canned or pouch-pack, 128
   Creamed Tuna with Noodles, 309
   Hot Tuna Wraps, 310
   Salad Niçoise, 195–96
   Tomatoes Stuffed with Curried Tuna
      Salad, 210
Turkey, 154, 265, 266
Turnips, 256, 290

Unsaturated fats, 100, 101, 102

Vanilla whey protein. *See* Whey protein
   powder
Vasopressin, 73
Vege-Sal, 142
Vegetables. *See also* Salads; Side dishes;
   specific kinds
   carbohydrates in, 37
   convenience foods, 127–28, 129–30
   glycemic indexes' misrepresentation of,
      45–47
Vegetarian recipes. *See also* Side dishes
   Apple-Walnut Pancakes, 180–81
   Apricot-Mustard Dressing, 213
   Balsamic-Mustard Sauce, 204
   Breakfast Cereal Sundae, 166
   Breakfast Custard, 163
   Cinnamon, Flax, and Bran Granola,
      175–76
   Classic Unpotato Salad, 205
   Coleslaw, 203
   Colorful Dill Egg Salad, 211
   Colorful Herb Frittata, 155–56
   Easy Pea Salad, 206
   Eggs Puttanesca, 162
   Flax Pancakes, 178
   Fruit Salad with Poppy Seed Dressing,
      209
   High-Fiber Bran Muffins, 173–74
   Hot "Cereal," 177
   Huevos el Diablo, 189
   Middle Eastern/Southwestern Fusion
      Salad, 207
   Molly's Piquant Onion Relish, 197
   Native American Flapjacks, 179
   Savory Scramble, 161
   Sort-of-Indian Omelet, 159
   Spiced Peanuts, 187
   Spinach-Mushroom Frittata, 152–53
   Spring-in-the-Wintertime Scramble, 160
   Strawberry Salad, 202